Traditional Chinese Therapeu

GW00393131

The Mystery of Longevity

Liu Zhengcai

Foreign Languages Press   Beijing

First Edition 1990
Third Printing 1996

Translated by Ouyang Caiwei

ISBN 7-119-01251-7

© Foreign Languages Press, 1990

Published by Foreign Languages Press
24 Baiwanzhuang Road, Beijing 100037, China

Distributed by China International Book Trading Corporation
35 Chegongzhuang Xilu, Beijing 100044, China
P.O. Box 399, Beijing, China

Printed in the People's Republic of China

CONTENTS

Preface

The way to good health and longevity has always been an intriguing topic for all peoples. In China the art of healthy living has evolved through thousands of years into a national tradition. It finds its way into history books, novels, stories, poems, Buddhist, Daoist, and Confucian classics, as well as numerous medical works. It is not surprising that every generation boasts a considerable number of centenarians. According to *The Yellow Emperor's Canon of Medicine* (*Huang Di Nei Jing*), people should "expend their naturally endowed life spans and pass away only after the age of a hundred."

An expert in traditional Chinese medicine from Sichuan Province, Liu Zhengcai has long been studying the art of longevity. Years ago he published *Essays on Healthy Living and Longevity*, which has received wide acclaim and appreciation from people both in China and abroad. His new book, *The Mystery of Longevity*, summerizes and expounds the secrets of Chinese centenarians over a period of several thousand years, such as conformity to nature, optimism, altruism, body-building exercises, methods for self-treatment, and food therapy.

Cao Cao (155-220), a famous statesman and villain-hero in Chinese history, declared in a poem,

> *Of one's earthly years*

Heaven gives no exact number;
Freedom from stress and sorrow
Will make one live longer.

No one can live forever, but a life span of a hundred years is within the reach of almost anyone who practises the traditional Chinese art of healthy living. Drawing on materials both ancient and modern, Liu Zhengcai has examined this field with commendable validity. Therefore I deem it a pleasure to preface his book.

Chen Keji
Professor of Geriatrics and Cardiology
at the China Academy of
Traditional Chinese Medicine

Introduction

Longevity is attainable, and a life span of a hundred years is no fiction. You will agree to this after you have been introduced by this book to numerous ancient Chinese centenarians mentioned in folklores, history books and documents, as well as to hundreds of centenarians who distribute throughout the country today.

What is the secret of longevity in terms of traditional Chinese medical theory? Based on ancient classics and county annals, the author has formulated a positive answer: "Go by the laws of yin and yang, do body-building exercises best suited to one's conditions, practise temperance in food and drink, follow a regular schedule in daily life, avoid overexertion, and keep calm and cheerful." All the points are illustrated with concrete examples. The emphasis on the relevance of wisdom and virtue to longevity, an ancient view confirmed by Confucius, shows the author's adherence to Chinese tradition.

Investigating into data about centenarians from China's third national census in 1982, the author sums up the experiences of urban centenarians, mostly intellectuals, into the following issues: regular physical labour; body-building exercises, brain usage and dedication to work; strict daily regimen; rational diet; clean and beautiful environment. He also accentuates family harmony and filial piety as the key to health and longevity in rural

China.

Traditional body-building exercises and medicines have always played a vital role in the everyday life of the Chinese people. This book provides the reader with body-building methods such as *daoyin* exercises, brocade exercises, games of five animals, and quiescent *qigong*. Also included are well-tried anti-senility medicines and favourite recipes of food therapy.

Most Chinese centenarians today are strong and healthy, thanks to their sound knowledge of traditional Chinese medicine and rich experiences in the prevention and self-treatment of common ailments. Therefore the book concludes with some simple methods for preventing and treating common ailments in the elderly.

Li Xiangfeng

Longevity in Ancient Chinese Centenarians

Chinese people have always cherished life, yearned for a long life span and accumulated experience in longevity since early antiquity. A unique way of preserving life was developed and thousands upon thousands of centenarians resulted. Books on how to preserve life and attain longevity are mentioned throughout China's historical records and more than three hundred titles remain extant.

Legend has it that quite a few ancient kings and political leaders known for their benevolent rule or military exploits lived more than a hundred years. Among them are Huang Di (Yellow Emperor), chief of the dominant clan in the Yellow River valley some five thousand to six thousand years ago who is now regarded as founder of the Chinese nation; Yao and Shun, both virtuous clan leaders who were later to be extolled by Confucianists as ideal sovereigns; Yu the Great of the Xia Dynasty (c. 21 cen. B.C.-c. early 16 cen. B.C.), who led his people to control the flood; King Tang, warrior-founder of the Shang Dynasty (c. early 16th cen. B.C.-c. 11th cen. B.C.); and several famous leaders in the Zhou Dynasty (11th cen. B.C.-256 B.C.), including Duke Zhou, held in great respect by Confucius as a model minister who served his sovereign properly.

Tradition says that famous ancient Chinese scholars enjoyed still longer life spans. For instance, Peng Zu, noted for his high skills in cuisine and the arts of *daoyin* and *qigong* in the times of Yao of Tang, lived to the age of seven hundred and sixty-seven when he went away without anybody knowing where. Lao Zi, author of the Daoist (Taoist) classic *The Canon of the Way* (*Dao De Jing*), reportedly lived three hundred years. A mysterious, rather shadowy figure in the Warring States Period (475 B.C.-221 B.C.) named Gui Gu Zi (Master of Ghost Valley) was said to have lived for several hundred years. He was highly skilled in body-building practices, meditation, and political and military strategy. As a true Daoist, he never dabbled in politics, but several of his disciples became distinguished statesmen serving in different rivaling states.

History has recorded personages of longevity in all dynasties, and they were especially numerous prior to the Jin Dynasty (265-420). In the reign of First Emperor of Qin (246 B.C.-210 B.C.), Cui Wen Zi, a Daoist good at caring for life, reportedly lived to the age of 300. In the period of Emperor Wu Di of Han, who rivaled the First Emperor in his intense interest in the way of immortality as well as in military exploits, a man named Li Gen of Xuxian County (present Xuchang County, Henan Province) was so well-versed in the secret of preserving life that he lived to be over 700. In the Eastern Han Dynasty (25-200), the famous physician Li Changzai wrote a book *Prescriptions of Li*, saying he could walk 800 *li* (400 kilometers) a day. He was popularly believed to have lived 800 years.

In the Three Kingdoms period (220 - 265) the villain-hero Cao Cao, ruler of the Kingdom of Wei, had three worthy scholars at his service. One of them was Gan Shi, a practitioner of higher skills of *qigong*. (A *qigong* practitioner attains the higher stage when he can make *qi* flow and circulate at will in his body. He undergoes unusual biological changes and can even walk on water or soar up into the sky.) Another was Zuo Ci, skilled in sexual techniques to make semen nourish the brain. The third was Xi Jian who could "dispense with cereals and only take *fuling* (*Poria cocos*, a subterranean fungus) as food." Well-known among their contemporaries for the art of preserving life, they each lived 300 years or more.

In the Jin Dynasty, a Handan native named Wang Lie looked young in his old age because he often ate sealwort (*rhizome polygonati*). Later he went into the Taihang Mountains to take ascetic religious training. He also lived to the age of 300.

It is impossible to discuss all such personages of longevity. Ge Hong (284 - 364), famous alchemist in the Jin Dynasty, wrote a book *Stories of Immortals* (*Shen Xian Zhuan*) in which he described ninety-four personages of longevity well-known in folklore and legend.

Of course, legends of those who lived several hundred years may not be too reliable, but there have indeed been a considerable number of authentic centenarians throughout China's history.

The blind court musician Grandpa Dou (350 B.C. - 170 B.C.) of the Western Han Dynasty lived to the age of 180. When asked by Han Emperor Wen Di about the secret of his longevity, Grandpa Dou replied that when he became blind at the age of thirteen his parents taught him the arts of *daoyin* and lute playing. Apart from this he had no other secret. The topic was picked up by Ji

Kang, one of the so-called Seven Sages of the Bamboo Grove in the Jin Dynasty, in his book *Preserving Life*. He said, "Grandpa Dou lived to the age of a hundred and eighty without taking any special tonics or nourishing foods or doing any particular body-building exercises. Didn't he achieve this because he felt tranquil from lute playing, which brought harmony to his mind? This is a way of nurturing the mind." Ji Kang suggests that music gave Grandpa Dou a long life.

Prime Minister Zhang Chang (? - 152 B.C.), during the reign of Han Emperor Wen Di, often drank human milk and is said to have lived more than a hundred years.

Hua Tuo, a celebrated physician in the late Eastern Han Dynasty, was the first in the world to use anaesthesia in surgery. According to *History of the Later Han Dynasty* (*Hou Han Shu*), "He had the looks of one in the prime of life when he was almost a hundred years old."

A historical record says that Leng Shouguang, a contemporary of Hua Tuo versed in body-building exercises and the art of healthy living, was as ruddy-cheeked as a man of thirty or forty when both his hair and beard had turned white. He lived to be over 150.

In addition, Huangfu Long, Feng Junda and Kuai Jing also lived more than a hundred years. Cao Cao received from Feng Junda, popularly known as the Youthful Daoist, a twenty-character life-preserving formula. It goes, "Exercise the body frequently, eat little, worry less, avoid excessive joy and anger and be temperate in sexual behaviour."

The Yellow Emperor's Canon of Medicine (*Huang Di Nei Jing*), the earliest medical classic in China, was written in the Warring States period and continuously supplemented by medical scientists in the Qin and Han dynasties. The book eloquently summarizes the longevity experiences of ancient centenarians. It says, "People well acquainted with the Way in remote times followed the principles of yin and yang, practised body-building exercises best suited to their own conditions, were temperate in food and drink, maintained a strict regimen in daily life and did not overexert themselves. That is why they remained in a good physical and mental state, enjoyed naturally endowed life spans and died only after the age of a hundred."

This unravels the mystery of longevity of ancient centenarians and represents the essence of the traditional Chinese way of caring for life. Among people of later generations who followed this way of caring for life, quite a few lived to be centenarians. Each of these personages and scholars had something to say about longevity from his own practical experience. A distinctive Chinese art of preserving life thus gradually evolved.

A close description of this unique art follows, based on the methods outlined in *The Yellow Emperor's Canon of Medicine* and supplemented on specific items by longevity experience of ancient Chinese centenarians and other creditable writings on the topic.

Follow the Principles of Yin and Yang

"Following the principles of yin and yang" means adapting oneself to environmental, especially climatic changes. Ancient scholars on the art of healthy living stressed preservation of life by adapting oneself to the changes of the four seasons. Their writings advanced the belief that if one adjusts oneself properly to climatic changes, one can enjoy good health and a long life. Ill-adaptation to external changes will result in diseases and a short life. A description is given below about how to preserve life in spring, summer, autumn and winter as recommended by ancient centenarians.

Caring for life in spring: With the rise of the spring sun, trees and grass are sprouting. In the second lunar month (from March to April) the weather turns warmer, but is still chilly. Weather changes in early spring easily bring relapses of former ailments in elderly people. As weather is sometimes warm and other times cold, it is inadvisable for old people to suddenly dispense with their cotton-padded clothes. They should remove their garment layers one by one. As they are weak and susceptible to the combined exopathogenic attack of wind and cold, they ought to have fine woollen knitwear or jackets with lining on hand at all times and put them on when the weather turns cool and take them off when it gets warm.

In spring days of warm sunshine and gentle breezes old people must not sit drowsily at home all day long because this easily leads to depression. Out in the country, flowers vie with one another in a riot of colours and young willow branches are sprouting and turning green. Old folks should go out on spring excursions to scenic spots and gardens, walk leisurely along a dyke or boat on a lake, sing or dance, listen to birds in the woods; this will make them feel delightful and brim with vitality.

Caring for life in summer: In summer the sun is scorching and the heat stifling. Old people weak in physique and vital energy will find it difficult to take good care of themselves. They should get up at early dawn when the air is refreshing, practise deep breathing exercises to exhale stale air and inhale fresh air, do traditional Chinese boxing and *daoyin* exercises.

On the hottest days old folks should not enjoy the cool under eaves, in corridors, at entrances to alleys, or at windows where wind blows strong. Although these places are cool, the drafts there are severely pathogenic. It suits an old person to rest in an empty hall, a quiet, clean room or a clear, spacious spot such as a waterside pavilion or shady woods where he will naturally remain cool. Moreover, he should regulate his breathing and keep his heart at peace so as to feel at all times as if ice and snow were refreshing his heart. He should not become irritated by the heat, for that only makes the heat more unbearable for him. People describe this as "a marvellous way to avoid summer heat. One does not need woods or a stream. Just rest calmly without any perplexing thoughts and one will arrive at refreshing mountains." In other words, "When one's heart is at peace, one will naturally feel cool."

Elderly people suffer from insufficiency of the yang of the spleen and stomach so they had better not eat ice or take cold drinks in summer months. They should also avoid eating anything raw, cold or greasy. Otherwise they may vomit and suffer from diarrhoea and this will impair their vitality and vigor and aggravate their weakness and fatigue. They may take green bean soup and dark plum drink to quench their thirst and refresh themselves in the heat.

It is inadvisable for old people to sleep under stars and moonlight in the open air. When sleeping, an old person should not stay in the breeze and should not ask somebody to fan him. Otherwise, wind will penetrate his body through pores and cause numbness of hands and feet. He should also, to prevent sunstroke, avoid working or walking in the scorching sun.

Caring for life in autumn: The weather turns cool in autumn, with sharp temperature differences between day and night. Ill-adapted to such weather changes, an old person could easily have a relapse of former ailments and contract new diseases. He should be ready at all times to add or take off clothes, and should do massage and *daoyin* exercises to limber up his tendons and joints and build his physique to guard against diseases.

At the Double Ninth Festival (the ninth day of the ninth lunar month) when the sky is clear and the air crisp and refreshing, an old person may stroll outside the city, climb hills to enjoy the surrounding scenery, compose poems by the waterside, take a short rest in the maple woods, gather chrysanthemums under the eastern hedge, or sing to the accompaniment of music. He should not be depressed by the sight of leaves falling in autumn wind, but should find inspiration in the famous line by the Tang poet Du Mu: "Frosty maples are redder than spring flowers."

In the droughty autumn air old people's blood and body fluids become dry and they often suffer from constipation. It suits them to eat sesame seeds, honey and similar food to nourish blood and body fluid and lubricate the intestines. They must avoid glutinous, hard, raw or cold foods to prevent autumn dysentery.

Caring for life in winter: Winter weather is cold in its world of ice and snow. It is advisable for the elderly to go to bed early and not get up until sunrise, thus avoiding cold by resting until the day warms up. An old person should gradually add clothes, and put on cotton-padded clothing only when the weather has become severely cold. It is inexpedient to wrap oneself in heavy woollen sweaters and cotton-padded garments when the weather is just beginning to turn cold. Otherwise, the body cannot stand up to weather changes when it becomes colder. The elderly should not sit at the fireside all day long, and if the bedroom is heated with a stove, special attention must be given to ventilation to guard against gas poisoning.

An old person must not sit quietly indoors in winter months. It is better to practise shadow boxing and fencing, exhale stale air and inhale fresh air, do *daoyin* exercises to limber up joints in the sunshine, tend trees and flowers or appreciate the snow and plum blossoms. These outdoor activities make a person warm and comfortable all over his body, generating feelings of spring and vitality despite the years. If one feels like dead ashes and curls up on bed or sits drearily, it will be more difficult to resist the cold.

In winter, it suits the elderly to eat warm, soft, well-cooked food, but not any tonic herbal or animal-based medicine hot in nature because in winter old people have internal heat, though they may be cold externally. Tonic medicines hot in nature will boost internal heat and cause inflammation. An old person can only take appropriate tonics warm in nature and drink a small glass of medicinal wine mornings and evenings to promote blood circulation and help resist cold.

The above-mentioned ways of preserving life in the four seasons are all practices of ancient people to adapt themselves to climate changes: the warmth of spring, the heat of summer, the chill of autumn and the cold of winter. Besides food, clothing, shelter and transportation, the Chinese put special emphasis on "nurturing the mind." One will naturally remain fit if one is always lighthearted, optimistic and willing to improve.

To enjoy tranquility and cheerfulness, one can take trips outside the city and visit mountains and streams in all seasons. In the Song Dynasty (960-1279) a man named You Shitai, who lived in Changzhou, was offered an office in the Imperial Academy of Learning. He declined because official duties would hinder him from travelling widely in preservation of his life. He visited famous mountains and rivers in all seasons and lived to the age of 120 to "die without any ailment."

The Yellow Emperor's Canon of Medicine states that a beautiful environment with fertile land and clear water is beneficial to longevity; this is supported by concrete examples in other classical writings. In the Jin Dynasty (265-420) a great Daoist alchemist named Ge Hong, who styled himself Master Baopu (Embracing Simplicity), was believed to be an immortal. His *Canon of Master Bao Pu (Bao Pu Zi)* records that Sweet Valley in Lixian County, Nanyang Prefecture abounded in chrysanthemums. Water in the valley tasted sweet and all local inhabitants drank water of the valley and, without exception, enjoyed long life spans.

Referring to the same valley, a famous geographer named Li Daoyuan (?-A.D. 527) of the Northern Wei said in *Commentary on the "Waterways Classic"*, "Chrysanthemum plants grow all along the headwaters and water in the streams and creeks are unusually delicious. It is said that this valley's water and soil are beneficial to good health and, drinking the water, people achieve longevity."

A more detailed description appears in *Geography of the Ming Empire* (*Ming Yi Tong Zhi*). "The water of the valley weighs more heavily than that of an islet. Sweet chrysanthemums grow beside the valley and the water was unusually sweet and fragrant. People in dozens of households lived more than a hundred just by drinking the water." But when some of the inhabitants moved elsewhere, they no longer attained the age of a hundred.

The close relation between longevity and natural environment is also testified by the existence of longevity areas. Hepu County in Guangxi Province features dense forests with towering ancient trees and clear streams where birds, beasts and fish flourish, favoring the inhabitants with a mild climate and abundant products. No wonder it has been a home of longevity since ancient times.

Su Dongpo (1037-1101), a famous poet and prose writer of the Northern Song Dynasty, said in *An Account of the Words of Hepu Oldsters*, "During my stay in Hepu, an eighty-one-year-old man named Su Foer visited me. He had two elder brothers, one aged ninety-two and the other ninety." There was also a man named Liu Jing who was born in 1085 and died at the age of 118 without any ailment. *The Annals of Lianzhou Prefecture* records that Hepu had seven centenarians in 1833. The 1982 national census showed that Hepu had thirteen centenarians among its 850,000 inhabitants.

The great benefit of favorable environment to health and longevity partly accounts for the building of Chinese Buddhist monasteries and Daoist temples in deep mountains with clear streams. Many Buddhist monks and Daoist priests living in such environments were centenarians. Among the famous Daoists who achieved longevity there were Xuanyuan Ji of Luofu Mountain, Guangdong; Chen Shu of Shantan Temple; Chen Yunsheng of Longhu Mountain in the Tang Dynasty. In the Song Dynasty there were Ding Shaowei of Huashan Mountain, Su Dengyin of Zhending Temple; and in the Ming Dynasty, Liu Yefu in Qingzhou and Yang Ruzhen in Fuzhou. All of them lived more than a hundred years. Buddhist monasteries also produced quite a few centenarians. For instance, a celebrated monk named Hui Zhao of the Tang Dynasty was born in 526 and died at the age of 290 in 816.

Of course, these people achieved longevity not only by living in a favorable environment, but also by practising meditation and body-building exercises.

Body-Building Exercises Best Suited to One's Conditions

Body-building exercises such as *daoyin*, *qigong* and massage are at the core of the Chinese art of preserving life. Ancient Chinese already realized that life lies in motion. *Lü's Almanac (Lü Shi Chun Qiu)*, compiled in the late Warring States period, states, "Running water is never stale and a door-hinge never gets worm-eaten. So it is with man's physique and vital energy." The great physician Sun Simiao (581-682) of the Tang Dynasty also remarked, "Running water is never stale and a door-hinge never gets worm-eaten. That is because they are in constant motion."

Chinese body-building exercises differ from Western-style sports in two respects. The Chinese creed of temperance and propriety is also applied to physical culture. Strenuous exercises should be avoided; one should not overexert oneself, but should do the kind and amount of exercises best fitted to one's ability and condition. Second, while strengthening one's physique, one should also learn to concentrate one's mind, either to direct *qi* to circulate in the body or to achieve a mental tranquility that brings one in harmony with Nature.

In ancient times quite a number of people lived to the age of 100 because they practised body-building exercises best fitted to their own conditions. Peng Zu, a legendary figure of about four thousand years ago, was believed to have lived for 800 years. His longevity was attributed to his practice of *qigong* and *daoyin* exercises. Zhuang Zi (369 B.C.-286 B.C.), a great Daoist philosopher, gave some description of the body-building exercises, though he did not approve of them, thinking that they would direct one away from the effort to attain true enlightenment. "Breathe deeply, fast and slow in turn; expel the old breath and take in the new; practise games in imitation of the movements of bears and birds —all this simply shows a desire for longevity. These practices are cherished by people who manipulate their breath and nourish their body, hoping to live as long as Peng Zu."

Xu Xun of the Jin Dynasty, who resigned as an official to become a physician, was also a regular practitioner of *daoyin* exercises. He was called Xu the True Master and lived to the age of 136. His art of *daoyin* exercises was later summarized into a widely popular book called *Miraculous Swordsmanship* (*Ling Jian Zi*). Wu Pu, a disciple of the famous physician Hua Tuo, persisted in practising the "games of five animals" that Hua Tuo had devised in imitation of the movements of tiger, deer, bear, ape and bird. He lived with good vision and hearing and firm teeth into his nineties.

A greater number of people practised *qigong* over a long time and became centenarians. Wu Dan of Liyi in the Jin Dynasty lived to be 170 by practising the higher skills of *qigong*. Daoist centenarian priests Ding Shaowei, Chen Shu, Chen Yunsheng, Su Chengyin, Liu Yefu and Yang Ruzhen were all known for their superb skills in *qigong*.

Every generation boasted a number of people who attained longevity by practising traditional martial arts such as limbering-up exercises for the tendons. The invention of limbering-up exercises for the tendons is generally attributed to Bodhidharma, the 28th Indian patriach in a direct line from Gautama Buddha who came to China in 520 to found the Chan (Zen) school of Buddhism in Shaolin Monastery, Henan. Very little is known about Bodhidharma's life, but history has it that by practising such exercises his disciple Hui Ke lived more than 100 years.

Higher skills in martial arts helped quite a few historical figures achieve longevity as well as military exploits.

Jagu Wulib served under Aguda, founder of the Jin regime, and was granted the title Duke of Rui. He lived 105 years.

Zabarhoch, a military commander who helped Genghis Khan found the Yuan Dynasty, lived to be 118.

Sun Yu, a successful candidate of martial arts in imperial examinations in the Ming Dynasty, had spent fourteen years guarding the frontier and died at 100.

Gong Laifu, a native of Guangzhou in the Ming Dynasty, was appointed senior commander of the Imperial Guards for his military exploits. He died at 138 when he was executed by Emperor Wu Zong for discouraging the emperor from going on an excursion.

Of those who achieved longevity through massage, Leng Qian of the Ming Dynasty was the most well-known. Apart from practising massage and *daoyin* exercises regularly, he loved music and was sort of a composer. He lived more than 150 years. His art of preserving life was summarized into *The Essentials of Achieving Longevity (Xiu Ling Yao Zhi)*, which contains "sixteen guidelines for preserving life," "eight methods for eliminating diseases" and "brocade exercises in twelve forms."

Temperance in Food and Drink

Temperance in food and drink is another secret for ancient centenarians. This include eating little, following a mainly vegetarian diet, drinking tea, paying attention to what one should abstain from in food and drink, and taking herbal and animal-based medicines.

Eating little: *The Yellow Emperor's Canon of Medicine (Huang Di Nei Jing)* says, "When one doubles his amount in food and drink, his stomach and intestines will be impaired," declaring that overeating impairs the functions of the stomach and intestines. Zhang Hua of the Jin Dynasty (265-420) wrote in his book *Records of Investigation of Things (Bo Wu Zhi)*: "The less one eats, the broader his mind, and the longer his life span; the more one eats, the narrower his mind, and the shorter his life span."

Ao Ying of the Ming Dynasty listed in his book *Random Words in East Valley* (*Dong Gu Zhui Yan*) the harm of overeating: "People who overeat will suffer from five physical disorders: First, frequent defecation; second, frequent urination; third, sleep disturbance; fourth, a body too heavy for exercise; and fifth, indigestion from taking in more than can be absorbed." In other words, overeating will make people grow fat and lead to other diseases. Consequently, Ao Ying advised people to eat less; but to what extent? Gong Tingxian, an imperial physician in Ming times, mentioned in his book *Disease Prevention to Achieve Longevity* (*Shou Shi Bao Yuan*):

"Eat to be only half full, and of no more than two dishes;

Drink seldom, and then only three tenths of one's capacity."

Ancient books contain many records of centenarians who maintained good health on limited amounts of food. Youthful Daoist who lived to be 100 also advised people that "one should always eat a limited amount of food." Centenarian physician Sun Simiao (581-682) wrote in his *Bedside Rhymes* (*Zhen Shang Ji*),

"A bowl of porridge in early morning,
Avoid a full meal at supper."

He indicated that "eating too full, after all, will not be beneficial." He also believed that frequent light meals would benefit elderly people while too much food and drink at a meal would impair their health.

A mainly vegetarian diet: Ancient scholars on the art

of healthy living consistently advocated taking plain food and avoiding rich, greasy meals; that is, adhering to a mainly vegetarian diet. When the centenarian Daoist Xuanyuan Ji of the Tang Dynasty replied to the inquiry of Emperor Wu Zong, he credited "taking plain food" for his longevity. Most Buddhist monks in monasteries and temples follow vegetarian diets so there are a fairly large number of long-lived men among the monks. The "List of Birth and Death Dates of Eminent Monks in Different Dynasties" records: Of 571 monks, 12 lived more than 100 years, 42 exceeded 90, 142 exceeded 80, 361 exceeded 70 and 433 exceeded 65, for a total of 75.8% living more than 65 years. Percentage of eminent monks living beyond the age of 65 was ten times that of emperors.

Zhu Danxi (1281-1385), a medical scientist of the Yuan Dynasty (1271-1368), advised in *Benefits of Plain Food on Health (Ru Dan Lun)* to follow mainly a vegetarian diet and to eat meat and vegetables in appropriate proportions. He advocated eating mainly "grains, beans, vegetables and fruit" and a limited amount of meat, cautioning that one should not eat more meat than vegetables. Too much meat regularly impairs the health and shortens life.

Drinking tea: China is the home of tea, where the habit of tea drinking has been popular ever since the fourth century. Lu Yu (733-804) of the Tang Dynasty wrote *The Canon of Tea (Cha Jing)*, China's (and the world's) first book on tea. Tea drinking was introduced to Japan in the ninth century and spread to Europe in the seventeenth century.

Ancient Chinese realized that tea drinking is of much benefit to health. *Shen Nong's Materia Medica (Shen*

Nong Ben Cao Jing), a book on medicinal herbs compiled in the Qin or Han dynasties, records, "Tea tastes bitter and to drink it improves the mind, dispels laziness, enlivens the body and brightens the sight."

Su Dongpo, a great poet and prose writer of the Northern Song Dynasty, advised people not to take medicine for minor ailments, but to drink tea. He wrote in a poem:

"Why is it necessary to take the elixir of immortals?
You may as well drink seven cups of tea as Lu Tong advised."

Lu Tong was a man of letters in Tang times noted for his dedication to tea drinking. He vividly described the marvels of drinking seven cups of tea:

"First cup moistens mouth and throat;
Second cup dispels loneliness and boredom;
Third cup makes the brain quick and lively,
capable of writing five thousand volumes;
Fourth cup brings mild perspiration,
draining all lifelong grievances through the pores.
Fifth cup refreshes muscles and bones;
Sixth cup brings communion with immortals;
No sooner has one drunk the seventh cup,
than a cool breeze lifts one up from below one's arms."

The poem gives a full account of the functions of tea. First, promoting saliva secretion and quenching thirst; second, making one strong and exhilarated; third, helping digestion and dissolving greasy food; fourth, inducing perspiration and curing common colds; fifth, reducing weight; sixth, invigorating thinking and strengthening memory, and seventh, prolonging life. When one has drunk the seventh cup, one feels as light as if one had broken the bonds of this world and become a winged immortal.

In the Song Dynasty, a Japanese monk named Ei Sai (1141-1245) who had come to study in China in 1187 wrote the book *Drinking Tea to Maintain Health* after returning to Japan. The book indicates that drinking tea is "the miraculous way to prolong life." A monk, aged 130, coming from Luoyang in 849, was asked by the emperor what medicines made him live so long. The monk replied he was very poor in his early youth and had no knowledge of the nature of medicinal herbs so he had not taken any medicine; yet he was fond of drinking tea in ordinary times. Accordingly, Emperor Xuan Zong bestowed twenty-five kilograms of tea leaves on him and appointed him abbot of Maintain-Longevity Monastery.

Abstinence from certain foods and drinks: Ancient scholars on the art of healthy living were careful to identify what one should avoid. Zhang Zhongjing, a celebrated physician of the Three Kingdoms period (220-265), listed in his book *Synopsis of Prescriptions of the Golden Chamber* (*Jin Gui Yao Lue*) what is best avoided from among birds, animals, fish and insects as well as fruits, grains and vegetables. He emphasized mainly that one should neither eat putrid food nor the meat of animals that had died of disease, advising people to pay attention to dietary hygiene.

The Confucian classic *Analects* (*Lun Yu*) records that Confucius "did not eat what was discoloured, what was of a bad flavour or what was ill-cooked," nor of "fish or meat that had become putrid or spoiled."

Jia Ming, a centenarian in the early Ming Dynasty, was specialized in the studies of food and drink people should avoid, and summerized his findings in *Essential Knowledge in Food and Drink (Yin Shi Xu Zhi)*. When Ming Emperor Tai Zu asked him the secrets for preserving life, he replied he had no secrets, except for paying attention to what he should not eat or drink, offering his book to the emperor. Jia Ming lived to the age of 106.

Giving up smoking and temperance in liquor were identified by ancient Chinese as essential for retaining good health. Tobacco was probably introduced into China in the early Ming Dynasty (1368-1644). At first people believed tobacco could cure diseases, but Lan Mou (1397-1446), a pharmacologist of the time, indicated in his book *Outline of Herb Medicine in Southern Yunnan (Dian Nan Ben Cao)* that tobacco was too hot and peppery and highly toxic.

Medical scientists of the Qing Dynasty (1644-1911) believed smoking was poisonous, making one "die of vomiting yellow fluid." Realizing the danger of addiction to smoking, Wu Yiluo in the Qian Long reign (1736-1795) said, "Smoking burns the yin of the lungs, causing people to suffer from sore throat and pharynx. Spitting blood and the loss of voice are common cases, which often result from addictive smoking. It consumes the blood and shortens the life span. Those concerned about their health should keep away from it."

A physician named Zhao Xuemin used a practical example to explore the dangers of smoking. His friend Zhang Shouzhuang suffered from coughing and spitting phlegm because of smoking, "taking medicine for over a year without effect." But, after giving up smoking for one month, both the cough and the phlegm cured themselves and "he was at once full of vigour and his appetite doubled." Consequently, Zhao concluded that smoking consumes the lungs and blood, impairs the spirit and shortens life. People should strive to abstain from the habit.

A book entitled *Give Up Smoking* published in the Qing Dynasty recommends steaming four ounces of perforated raw bean curd topped by two ounces of brown sugar until the sugar melts, and drinking the sweetened bean curd juice to defeat the urge to smoke. It was said that one would banish the urge to smoke after taking the recipe for three days.

Wine and liquor have a long history in China. In remote times people used wine or liquor to treat ailments. Later, some became habitual, excessive drinkers and alcohol became an important factor in causing disease. For instance, *Lü's Almanac* (*Lü Shi Chun Qiu*) says, "Heavy drinking is the ringleader in occurrence of diseases." But drinking a limited amount of liquor is beneficial to the human body. Husehui, an imperial physician of the Yuan Dynasty, analyzed the benefits and harms of liquor in his book *Essentials in Food and Drink* (*Yin Shan Zheng Yao*), a book on nutrition and cuisine: "Liquor ... brings the function of medicinal herbs into full play in the human body, eliminates all evils, promotes blood circulation, nourishes stomach and intestines and dissipates worries. Therefore, if one drinks a limited amount of liquor, it keeps him in good health. Excessive drinking impairs the mind, shortens the life span and changes one's intrinsic nature."

All physicians of later generations have believed that drinking a limited amount of liquor can promote blood circulation and limber muscles and tendons, but that excessive drinking is harmful. Consequently, veteran traditional Chinese physicians like to drink some liquor, but few drink excessively.

Medicinal liquor brewed with life-prolonging medicinal herbs and mountain springs can help people attain longevity. For example, a family on Funiu Hill often drank a liquor brewed with medicinal herbs and a five-vent spring. The old man lived to the age of 140 and his eldest son 123.

Certainly, when discussing food and drink to avoid, emphasis should always be placed on avoiding salty food. Dangers of too much salt were discovered early. Sun Simiao indicated in *Maxims for Preserving Life* (*Bao Sheng Ming*), "Food that is too salty shortens the life span. Do not show preference to such food."

Notes on Preserving Life (*Yang Sheng Fu Yu*) written by Chen Jiru of the Ming Dynasty recorded that three elderly men "are all in their eighties and in unusually good health." When asked about the cause, their answers were the same: "It is difficult to get salt here. We all eat light-flavoured food." Another man, Ma Jiantian, was robust and still had black hair and beard at the age of 65. He also attributed this to "eating little salt." So the Daoist book *Canon of Alchemy* (*Dan Shu*) says, "Eating food of light flavour refreshes one's mind." There is also a Chinese folk saying, "Rice and other dishes should be simple and light in flavour; little salt causes few ailments."

Herbal medicines: Some ancient centenarians often took tonic medicinal herbs. Meng Shen of the Tang Dynasty who wrote *Outline of Herb Medicine as Food Therapy* (*Shi Liao Ben Cao*) said, "To preserve the body and cultivate the mind, one should constantly say kind-hearted words and take good medicines."

Husehui of the Yuan Dynasty also advocated cooking medicinal herbs with food, calling it food therapy. His nutrition book *Essentials in Food and Drink* (*Yin Shan Zheng Yao*) records instances of people who took medicinal herbs as food and achieved longevity.

While making an inspection tour on Mount Tai in east China, Han Emperor Wu Di (156-87 B.C.), seeing an old man ploughing farmland on the roadside, asked about his age. The old man replied that his age was 180, adding that when he was 85 years old, his hair turned white, all his teeth fell out and he was extremely decrepit and on the verge of death. However, he met a Daoist priest who advised him to eat dates and drink only water, avoiding all other food and to sleep on a medicinal pillow. Before long he grew strong, his white hair turned black and new teeth grew in. Emperor Wu Di inquired of the man's neighbours and they verified his words.

Notes on Preserving Life (*Yang Sheng Fu Yu*) also talks of Daoist priests on Zhongnan Mountain who lived to ages between 100 and 200. The main reason for their longevity was digging up sealwort (*Polygonatum sibiricum*), the rhizome of Chinese atractylodes and the rhizome of large-headed atractylodes (*Atractylodes macrocephala*) for use as food.

Wang Lie, a native of Handan of the Jin Dynasty (265-420), often ate sealwort and looked young in his old age. He reportedly lived to be over 300. Yue Chang, a Daoist priest of Jimo (in present Shandong Province) in the Song Dynasty, remained in such good health his youthful countenance was at odds with his white hair.

He was still healthy at the age of 180 because he took, over a long period of time, longevity-promoting decoctions of herbal powder from black sesame and red beans, prepared from a special prescription.

Food recipes such as herbal porridge shall be dealt with in a special section later in the book.

A Regular Daily Regimen

One of the secrets of longevity of ancient centenarians was to live a regular life, to work and rest according to an established schedule.

Ancient scholars on the art of healthy living recognized the effect of work-and-rest habits on one's health and life span. In the Spirng and Autumn period Guan Zi (?-645 B.C.) indicated, "An irregular daily life ... will result in overfatigue and a shortened life span." Sun Simiao also said, "One who is good at preserving life gets up and goes to bed by a timetable adjusted to different seasons, and maintains a strict regimen in daily life." *The Canon of Medicine* prescribed a daily schedule adapted to climatic changes in the four seasons. Scholars in later generations worked out ways of preserving life by using the 12 *shichen* (two-hour periods) named after the Twelve Earthly Branches.

According to *The Canon of Medicine*, in spring "one should go to bed late and get up early and stroll in the courtyard"; in summer "one should go to bed late and get up early and keep doing body-building exercises without being afraid of sunshine"; in autumn "one should go to bed early and get up early, rising as soon as the cock crows," and in winter "one should go to bed early and get up late, awaiting warm sunshine." It said those who "drink excessive liquor, get up and go to bed at irregular hours and have sex when drunk," namely, people who do not observe a regular timetable in daily life, will become decrepit at the age of 50 and die before their time.

Caring for life in 12 *shichen*: The practice was referred to by the Daoist of Stone Chamber of the Ming Dynasty as "12-*shichen* exercises." You Cheng, a physician of the Qing Dynasty, called it "12-*shichen* disease-eliminating method." Here is a brief summary of the writings of various scholars on this topic.

The *mao* period (5-7 a.m.): At sunrise, get up and tap teeth together 300 times, swing shoulders back and forth to loosen muscles and tendons. Then rub hands until they are warm, massage both sides of the nose and both eyes six or seven times and rub and curl both ears five or six times. The next step is to place the palms of the hands over the ears, fingers on the back of the head, placing the forefingers on the middle fingers and tapping the back of the head with the forefingers of both hands 24 times each, an exercise called "beating the heavenly drum." Then go outdoors to do *daoyin* exercises.

The *chen* period (7-9 a.m.): After finishing *daoyin* exercises, drink a cup of boiling water or tea, then comb the hair with hands instead of a comb, doing it more than 100 times to refresh the mind and brighten vision. Then wash face and rinse mouth. Porridge or other light food are most suitable for breakfast, after which a slow walk for 100 paces while massaging abdomen with the hands benefits the spleen and promotes digestion.

The *si* period (9-11 a.m.): Read a book, do housework, grow vegetables or tend flowers. When tired, sit quietly to nourish the mind or tap the teeth together and swallow the saliva. Since the elderly are short of breath, it is better not to talk aloud with others for very long. Talk consumes *qi*, so it is best to "talk little to nourish *qi*."

The *wu* period (11 a.m.-1 p.m.): Eat to 80 percent of full at lunch, making sure to rinse mouth with tea to dissolve the grease. Then sit quietly for some time or take a nap.

The *wei* period (1-3 p.m.): Take a nap, practise *qigong*, play chess, read gazettes or do housework.

The *shen* period (3-5 p.m.): Read or write poems, practise calligraphy or painting, play the lute, go outdoors to gaze at sunset clouds, work for a short while in the fields or take a stroll on the pathways between fields.

The *you* period (5-7 p.m.): Practise *daoyin* exercises. Eat early and little for supper. It is all right to drink a small glass of spirituous liquor but take care not to get drunk. Rinse mouth and brush teeth before going to bed to remove residue and anything harmful to health and wash feet with warm water to reduce internal heat and promote blood circulation.

The *xu* period (7-9 p.m.): Practise *qigong* exercises and go to bed. It is best to "lie in the shape of a bow." Calm the mind before closing the eyes.

The *hai* and *zi* periods (9 p.m. to 1 a.m.): Curl up with bent knees in sleep, but when awake stretch, relax and shift to promote the circulation of *qi* and blood. Go to bed in a quiet environment and sleep tranquilly to nourish the *qi*.

The *chou* and *yin* periods (1-5 a.m.): These are the time when *jing* (essence) and *qi* begin to grow. As *jing* and *qi* are the very treasures of man, it is unadvisable to consume too much of them in sex, though excessive continence can also be harmful. Generally speaking, it is best for elderly people to have sex once every 20 to 30 days.

In ancient times most recluses, Daoist centenarians and those who had retired from official posts followed this schedule to stay healthy. For instance, Bai Juyi (772-846), a famous poet of the Tang Dynasty who retired to Fragrant Hills in Luoyang, Henan Province in his late years, spent his time with several celebrated oldsters, the youngest of whom was in his seventies. Oldest were Li Yuanshuang of Luozhong who lived to the age of 136 and Buddhist monk Ru Man who attained the age of 95. Not bothered with government affairs, they could maintain such a strict regimen to achieve longevity.

In many of his poems Bai Juyi described his life of leisure and discipline:

> "*Morning sunshine comes in to the eastern room,*
> *I tap my teeth together 36 times.*"
> "*At sunset I go out to look at the fields;*
> *Strolling up and down the village.*"
> "*Two simple vegetarian meals in morning and even-ing,*
> *An idle nap at mid-day.*
> *This is how I spend my days,*
> *I have lived in this way for three years.*"
> "*What am I doing all day long?*
> *Drink a cup of tea or compose two lines of poetry.*"

In his youth and prime, Bai Juyi suffered both from stomach trouble and eye ailment and was weak in constitution. Because he consistently maintained a strict regimen and took good care of himself, he turned out to be the longest lived of all famous Chinese poets, living to 74. According to "Seven Oldsters Meet to Compose Poems": "The seven of us add up to the age of 584." Their average age was at least 83 while the life span of people at that time was only 33. This illustrates that to live, work and rest according to a strict regimen, indeed, represents one of the secrets of longevity.

Among other things, the 12-*shichen* exercises advise one to get up and tap teeth 300 times in the *mao* period (5-7 a.m.) and again tap teeth and swallow saliva in the *si* period (9-11 a.m.). This keeps the teeth firm and durable and helps prolong life. Daoist priest Kuai Jing of the Three Kingdoms period (220-265) kept getting up early, tapping teeth together and swallowing saliva. He lived to the age of 178. Huangfu Long followed his example and also lived to be over 100.

Avoid Overexertion

Avoiding overexertion was another important way to care for life among ancient centenarians and one of the secrets of longevity. Ancient scholars on the art of healthy living advised against physical or mental over-exertion, especially sexual indulgence. As a major feature of Chinese tradition of preserving life, sexual temperance is here dealt with in detail.

The Canon of Medicine indicates, "Engaging in un-timely, improper or excessive sexual relations as a regular practice and having sexual relations when drunk will consume one's essence of life stored in the kidney," and this is one of the main causes of premature senility and declining health. Sun Simiao described this more vividly and fully 1,400 years ago:

"Kings and marquises keep several thousand beautiful ladies in their palaces and harems; high-ranking officials keep several hundred concubines in their mansions. They drink strong liquor to impair their marrow in daytime and consume their *qi* and blood in sexual performances at night. They indulge their ears in obscene sounds and their eyes in voluptuous sights.... If there are few centenarians today, is it not because these people behave improperly?"

All the scholars on the art of healthy living and medical scientists in later generations emphasize the significance of restraining sexual desires and being temperate in sexual behaviour, for sexual relations consume the *jing* in the kidney. When too much *jing* is drained from the kidney, life span will inevitably be affected. As *Simple Explanations of Medical Science on Healthy Living* (*Yang Sheng Yi Yao Qian Shuo*) indicates, "Those who keep the yang vigorous and preserve the *jing* from childhood to old age will attain longevity even if they are weak in constitution, while those who consume their *jing* and marrow day in and day out will inevitably have short lives, even if they are robust."

The ancients gave several advices on the preservation of *jing* to prolong life.

1. Late marriage. *The Book of Rites* (*Li Ji*, a Confucian classic) says men should not marry until the age of 30 and women should not marry until they are 20. Zhu Danxi, a medical scientist in the Jin (1115-1234) and Yuan dynasties, reiterated this opinion, vigorously advocating late marriage. Gong Tingxian, a physician in the

Ming Dynasty, described the harm of early marriage upon people's health: "If a man loses his virginity too early, this will impair the *jing* in the kidney; if a woman loses her virginity too early, this will impair her blood system."

2. Fewer children. Wang Chong, a philosopher and scholar on the art of healthy living in Han times, in *Discourses Weighed in the Balance* (*Lun Heng*) talked about women and child bearing: "When a woman bears few children, they survive; when she bears many, they die." It means if a woman marries late and bears few children, they will easily survive, while if she marries early and bears many children, they will often be short-lived.

3. Sex at regular intervals. In his book on how to preserve life and bear fine children, Wang Gui, a scholar on the art of healthy living in the Yuan Dynasty, indicated that it is best for people at the age of 30 to have sexual relations once every eight days and those at the age of 40 once every 16 days. Those at the age of 50 are declining in vigour and should have sexual relations once every 20 days and those at the age of 60 should refrain from sex, but if they find it difficult, once a month is suggested.

Ancient scholars on the art of healthy living believed that whoever was dissipated and indulged in sexual desires, violating the rules above, would be short-lived. Very few emperors enjoyed longevity mainly because of excessive dissipation. Of the more than 300 Chinese emperors since the Qin Dynasty (221 B.C.-206 B.C.), only eight exceeded 70, and none has been known to be a centenarian. Emperor Xian Feng of the Qing Dynasty indulged himself in women and songs all day long, dying early at the age of 30.

Therefore, all centenarian recluses restrained sexual desires and were temperate in sex. When emperors ask them about ways of preserving life, they always emphasized this point. Feng Junda, a centenarian Daoist priest of the Three Kingdoms period, advised Cao Cao to "avoid over-indulgence in sex." Xuanyuan Ji, a Daoist priest on Luofu Mountain of Tang times, also advised Tang Emperor Wu Zong to "keep away from women and songs." Su Chengyin, a centenarian Daoist priest of Song times, advised Song Emperor Tai Zu (927-976) to be "free of desires," namely to keep a tranquil mind, restrain sexual desires and be temperate in sexual behaviour. However, one cannot expect emperors to follow such an advice when they had several thousand maids of honour and hundreds of concubines in the palace. No wonder many of them came to a premature end.

Quite a number of ordinary people are known to have prolonged their lives by abstaining from sexual activity. *Notes on Preserving Life (Yang Sheng Fu Yu)* of the Ming Dynasty tells of Dong Sangang who, consistently weak in constitution, fathered a son at the age of 60. In order to raise his son to adulthood, he decided to "abstain from sexual desires to prolong life." He lived alone, sending his several concubines elsewhere, and lived to the age of 78.

Another man, Yan Jiexi, began abstaining from sex at the age of 40 and lived to the age of 85. *Maxims on Prolonging Life (Yan Shou Di Yi Shen Yan)*, written by Old Man of Stupid Valley of Song times, also records many successful efforts to prolong life by refraining from sex. Cheng Yichuan, a philosopher and educator of the same dynasty, had been weak in constitution since childhood. He became weaker after his marriage at the age of 30 and was decrepit and on the verge of death in his forties. Once he decided to abstain from sex, his physical health improved and he became robust. At the age of 72 he was stronger than at any other time in his life.

Keep Calm and Cheerful

The Canon of Medicine (*Nei Jing*) advises, in summing the experiences of centenarians in remote times: "Do not be weighed down by perplexing thoughts; strive to be calm and optimistic; be complacent; keep sound in body and mind. This way one can live to the age of 100."

The Canon of Medicine recognizes that emotional and psychological factors are important causes for illness. It indicates that excessive emotion impairs the internal organs of the human body. "Anger hurts the liver, joy hurts the heart, brooding hurts the spleen and melancholy hurts the lungs." Hence it proposes regulating the emotions by "keeping the heart calm and cheerful and the mind free of worries." "Where can diseases come from when the emotional state maintains inner composure?" Scholars on the art of healthy living in subsequent generations set forth many specific methods of maintaining optimism in accordance with this principle.

Shi Tianji, a scholar on the art of healthy living in the Ming Dynasty, proposed "Six Always" for maintaining a calm and cheerful state of mind:

Always be peaceful in mind. Remain peaceful in mind without vain hopes. Do not covet, do not indulge in vain wishes, do not worry about personal gains and losses. Hence Shi Tianji said, "If one has few desires, his mind will naturally be peaceful. Just look at secluded hills and remote valleys! Most people there enjoy long life spans because they have few desires and always remain peaceful in mind."

Always be kind-hearted. A kind-hearted person often takes pleasure in helping others and has no desire to harm others. Whenever he conceives an idea, makes a remark or does a deed, he always ponders whether it is beneficial or harmful to others. "When others are evil, I remain upright; when others are vicious, I remain kind-hearted; when others stir up troubles, I strive to alleviate troubles; when others harm people, I serve people. If I act in this way, I shall have a clear conscience and naturally feel calm and tranquil in mind."

Always uphold justice. Distinguish between evil and virtue and between right and wrong. Virtue and evil are antagonistic, and right and wrong are not to be confused. If one maintains his awareness, upholds integrity and remains clear-headed and sharp-eyed, he will naturally be free from worries and troubles. Hence Shi Tianji said, "Only when scholars are equipped with awareness will illusions and fantasies vanish. When the sun shines in the sky, obscurity is naturally cleared away. When one grasps this miraculous concept, he will be cured of disease and attain longevity as well."

Always be cheerful. Adapt to different circumstances; feel complacent at all times; avoid overdoing anything and do not hurt anyone's feelings. As Bai Juyi says in a poem:

Be cheerful, whether rich or poor,

He who does not laugh can only be a fool.

One should often have hearty laughs. A folk saying goes, "A good laugh makes one ten years younger; worry turns the hair gray."

Always be pleasant. Harmony is paramount in human relations. Be amiable, modest and prudent, broadminded and magnanimous; do not be calculating and do not worry about trifles. To be amiable in dealing with others will bring happiness to both the others and oneself.

Always be contented. It is a rare person who avoids all adversity. One should remain cheerful despite adversities. Yan Feitai had a wise epigram on caring for life. "Look forward, one thinks one possesses one thing but lacks another, that he is in short of this and that. Step back, one finds one can lead an easy life just by eating this bowl of porridge and wearing this garment." The first sentence refers to the distress of discontent and the second the joy of content. "Just step back to think, everything will naturally be all right." "Contentment is happiness." Whenever there is adversity, compare it with a worse circumstance and one will feel calm and cheerful.

Another scholar on the art of healthy living in the Ming Dynasty, Wang Xun'an, proposed "taking pleasure in the world" to remain cheerful and optimistic. Recognition of pleasure helps to maintain contentment. Here is a list of some simple pleasures.

The pleasure of sitting quietly. When one sits quietly for a short while after work, all worries are gone and one feels unhurried, carefree and relaxed. It is like a jar of muddy water: stir it all day long and it will be turbid throughout the day; allow it to be undisturbed for a moment and it will become clear and transparent.

The pleasure of reading. Reading is the happiest activity on earth; it makes one know more and understand better. It makes a foolish man virtuous and stupid man wise. When Confucius was reading he became so absorbed he forgot meals and so happy he forgot all worries and ignored that old age was advancing.

The pleasure of appreciating flowers. Peach and prune blossoms in spring, sweet osmanthus and chrysanthemums in autumn, lotus and plum flowers in summer and winter—one can feast on flowers in all four seasons. Chinese Rose is praised as the loveliest of all flowers. It blossoms often and is longlasting, providing pleasure throughout the four seasons. It can be called the "longevity flower." By planting flowers and trees around the house, one creats a pleasurable environment for oneself and will naturally feel happy and lighthearted.

The pleasure of appreciating the moon. All curio enthusiasts love tripods of the Zhou Dynasty and jades of Han times but these objects are not as antique as the moon. As the great poet Li Bai wrote,

People of today have not seen the ancient moon,
But today's moon once shone over the ancients.

Love of antiques cannot compare with appreciation of the moon. On a breezy, moonlit night, sing a song or compose a poem while gazing at the moon. One will be lost in a fairyland of boundless pleasure.

The pleasure of appreciating paintings. The best way to appreciate a painting is to imagine oneself in it —green hills and streams, flowers, birds, terraces and towers. Looking at a snowy scene makes one feel cool and refreshed in summer; a picture of summer scenery makes one feel warm and high-spirited in winter. Look at portraits to observe the expressions of characters; look at flowers, insects and fish to examine their postures and movements. There is boundless pleasure in identifying oneself with paintings. It is more gratifying, of course, if one can paint for oneself.

The pleasure of listening to bird song. Orioles sing and swallows dart to welcome spring. Hearing the call of birds in the woods always gives one much delight.

The pleasure of unrestrained singing and recitation. A poetry lover may intone his favorite poems on a mountain peak or beside a stream. This will make one feel happy and carefree and dispel all his worries.

The pleasure of appreciating landscape. Confucius said, "The wise find pleasure in water; the virtuous find pleasure in mountains." Magnificent landscapes and beautiful scenery on bright days are found here and there. One may find infinite pleasure while travelling over hills and beside streams. When one visits towers, pavilions, and terraces, one will recall the virtues and exploits of the ancients. One may gaze at high mountains and cloud-shrouded valleys. At the sight of happy, carefree fish one becomes happy too; among green trees and clear streams one becomes refreshed and pure. One's mind becomes as broad as the sky as he lives in harmony with Nature.

The pleasure of listening to or playing music. Plucking the strings of a lute gives one spiritual nourishment and hightens one's mind. When Confucius was in the State of Qi, he heard the Shao music and for three months did not know the taste of meat. Evidently, the music of lutes, bells and drums have a great power over one's soul. Music nourishes both mind and body and helps one achieve longevity.

The pleasure of dancing. Mencius (c. B.C.372-B.C. 289) said, "When they are rejoiced, they grow. Growing, how can they be repressed? When they come to this state that they cannot be repressed, then unconsciously the feet begin to dance and the hands to move." "On Ancient Music" in *Lü's Almanac* (*Lü Shi Chun Qiu*) refers to dancing as an important means of strengthening the physique, broadening the mind, regulating blood and *qi* and assuaging sorrow and melancholy.

Many ancient Chinese centenarians loved music, chess, calligraphy and painting. Grandpa Dou, whom we mentioned earlier, of Han times, reached the age of 180 because he played the lute and felt cheerful all day long. Leng Qian of the Ming Dynasty was versed in music as well as massage and lived to the age of 150. Guo Zhenshun, a woman poet of Chaozhou in Ming times, loved to compose poems and rhymed prose and lived to the age of 125. Lin Chunze, a Confucian scholar of the same dynasty, was steeped in the *Book of Rites* (*Li Ji*) and the art of writing poems and essays. Poetry made him hale and hearty both in body and mind and he lived to the age of 104. He Cheng, a native of Jiangyin County in Ming times, was a proficient painter of bamboo and rocks. He also lived to the age of 100.

Genetic Strength and Long Life

The Canon of Medicine says, "A person takes the mother as foundation and the father as shield." Wang

Chong, a philosopher of the Eastern Han Dynasty, declares, "A person is strong and long-lived or weak and short-lived. This depends on whether one is richly or poorly endowed in constitution by nature.... When richly endowed in constitution, he is strong in physique and long-lived. When poorly endowed in constitution, he is weak in physique and short-lived." *Notes on Preserving Life (Yang Sheng Fu Yu)* says, "Whether a person is fat or thin should be attributed to one's mother; whether a person lives long or short should be attributed to one's father." *Maxims on Prolonging Life (Yan Shou Di Yi Shen Yan)* records instances when men chose tall women as wives to have tall sons. Evidently, the ancients already recognized the importance of heredity in constitution and life span.

Precisely because of relationships between a person's life span and heredity, there were long-lived families and short-lived families in Chinese history. For instance, the family of Yang Biju, a native of Qiongzhou in Song times, produced eight or nine generations of centenarians. A prefect named Li, who called on the family, saw that Yang's several uncles were all in their 120s, his grandfather was more than 160 and still healthy, and Yang Biju himself was 100 years old.

Miscellaneous Notes of the Annals of Suzhou Prefecture (Su Zhou Fu Zhi Za Ji) records: "When Emperor Qian Long in the 16th year of his reign (1751) went on an inspection tour in the south, 140-year-old Tang Ercheng of Hunan Province came to welcome him.... All his accompanying great grandchildren were white-haired old men." When members of several generations in a family attained longevity, it should certainly be attributed to hereditary factors.

A scholar of the Qing Dynasty named Zhao Yi records in his notebook about a family of short-lived members: "Formerly Xie Zhuang said that none of his family members had had a long life span. His great great grandfather died at the age of 40, his great grandfather at the age of 32, his grandfather at the age of 47, and Xie Zhuang himself died at the age of 46."

However, the influence of heredity over a person's life span is by no wise absolute. Wang Chong proposed to compensate undesirable hereditary factors by what is now a method of improving the human species through selective mating to provide children with strengths of their parents.

Maxims on Prolonging Life (Yan Shou Di Yi Shen Yan) recommends careful choosing of spouses. According to traditional Chinese medical theory, if a person has poor congenital qualities from heredity, it is possible to improve this condition through intensive care after his birth. *Notes on Preserving Life* also says, "Whether a person lives long or short should be attributed to his father, ... but the cultivation of body, mind and lofty morals is his own responsibility." Consequently, provided a person pays attention to the art of healthy living, he can expect to attain longevity even if his parents are short-lived. For instance, Yu Minde, a native of Dinghai in Ming times, was orphaned at an early age. When grown up, he planted many bamboos and trees around his house and took good care of himself in daily life. He lived to the age of 105.

Apart from heredity, there is another important factor of family harmony and filial children. This is a fine Chinese tradition. Fathers should be affectionate, sons should be filial and a family should live in harmony. Sun

Simiao said, "In accordance with the principle of filial piety, one must take good care of one's aged parents." He also advised that "a filial son should be well-acquainted with the nature of food and medicine" in order to look well after his parents.

Gong Tingxian indicates in his *Secret Prescriptions of Prince Lu's Mansion (Lu Fu Jin Fang)*: "People should respect and act upon Confucius' instructions.... When children and grandchildren are filial, this prolongs the life of the elderly." He also advised that "father should be strict but not excessive in disciplining his children; mother should be affectionate but not over-solicitous; son should be filial to his parents without neglecting their wishes; wife should be virtuous and not jealous; elder brother should be kind and not arrogant; younger brother should be respectful without ignoring instructions of the elder. To achieve family harmony, there should be no vicious gossip; if a family wants to preserve its wealth, it should not divide up its property." If members of a family live together in harmony under one roof and look after one another affectionately in an amiable atmosphere, they can achieve longevity.

The ancients told many stories about how filial children achieved longevity together with their parents who received good care. Zhang Chuan, a native of Haining of Ming times, was learned, filial, and of high moral character. Local people recommended him as an official but he declined, saying he had to look after his mother. He stayed at home and took good care of his aged mother. His mother lived to the age of 99 and Zhang Chuan reached the age of 102. Both mother and son achieved longevity with a combined age of 200.

Li Shi, a teacher in Ruian in the Song Dynasty, was

filial to his parents all his life. His father died when he was already in his 90s. His mother was still alive at the age of 119.

Virtue and Long Life

According to *Analects*, Confucius once declared that "the virtuous live long." He also said, "Having such great virtue, ...one can surely attain longevity," meaning that those who have good moral characters will enjoy good health and long lives.

Mencius inherited and developed this Confucian theory and described the specifics of moral cultivation. A man of integrity "does not lose course when rich, faith when poor, or heart when subject to authority."

The Canon of Medicine also says that those "who are able to live their full life spans and die at the age of 100" have a perfect moral character and do not risk unnecessary danger.

Most medical scientists and scholars on the art of healthy living in later generations put moral cultivation paramount in preservation of life. Wu Pu, a disciple of Hua Tuo, said, "Those who are good at maintaining health should first eliminate six harms before they can preserve their lives and live to the age of 100. First, depreciate fame and wealth. Second, keep away from women and sensuous songs. Third, disdain merchandise and other material wealth. Fourth, ignore flavour in food and drink. Fifth, eliminate obsequiousness and arrogance. Sixth, free the self from jealousy." All the six points, except for the fourth, deal with moral cultivation.

Lü Shujian of Ming times says in his book *Moans and Groans (Shen Yin Yu)*, "Moral cultivation is of primary importance for the preservation of life." Shi Tianji also believes, "Those who are skilled at preserving life should stress moral conduct, coupled with the art of maintaining health. Both can be carried out without conflict. Thus, one will naturally become healthy and strong and live long."

Why can the virtuous live long? Dong Zhongshu (179 B.C.-104 B.C.), a great exemplifier of Confucianism in the Western Han Dynasty, says in his book *Spring and Autumn Studies (Chun Qiu Fan Lu)*: "The reason why the virtuous live long is that they are not greedy for outward gains and are able to keep inward peace. Their minds keep calm and tranquil and do not stray from the principle of integrity; but they assimilate the beauty of nature to preserve life."

Wang Wenlu, a scholar on the art of healthy living in the Ming Dynasty, also believes that the virtuous live long because those who prize moral cultivation remain tranquil in their minds and maintain untroubled will power. Their vitality and organisms are in harmony and blood in smooth flow. So they are not susceptible to diseases and naturally they are healthy and can live long.

The famous centenarian physician Sun Simiao of the Tang Dynasty was a typical example of the long life of the virtuous. He did not seek fame and wealth and was content with plain living. Sui Emperor Wen Di (541-604) appointed him to be an official of the Imperial Academy. Tang emperors Tai Zong (599-649) and Gao Zong (628-683) called him to the capital to appoint him to high-ranking position with handsome salaries. But he declined all these offers and devoted himself to medical studies. He was determined to relieve common people from diseases and ailments. He strove to improve his medical skills and treated patients as kith and kin. Whether they were rich and distinguished or poor and low, relatives, intimate friends or total strangers, they were treated equally without discrimination. If the patient could not come to see him he always went personally to see the patient regardless of weather or distance. He gave his patients all his attention and had little interest in money or material rewards. He neither showed off his learning and skills nor disparaged other physicians. Precisely because he had good moral character and lofty medical ethics and was skilled at the art of healthy living, he lived to the age of 101. According to one scholar, he actually attained the age of 141.

Most of the ancient centenarians were known for their virtue. For example, Lü Shixian of the Ming Dynasty was charitable and willing to help the poor, upright and chivalrous, often defended others against injustice and helped people who were in danger or financial difficulty. He had a good appetite, was fond of sports and manual work, walked with vigorous strides and lived to the age of 103. Fang Dequan, a native of Fenghua, Ningbo of Ming times, was industrious and plain living and often helped those in financial trouble. He was honest, kind-hearted and generous to people. Four generations of his family with some 100 members lived together in harmony under one roof. He reached the age of 100. ·

Wisdom and Long Life

"The wise live long" is a traditional Chinese view first affirmed and expostulated by Confucius. This can be found in *The Sayings of Confucius* (*Kong Zi Jia Yu*), a book compiled by Wang Su of the Three Kingdoms period. Duke Ai of the state of Lu asked Confucius, "Do the wise live long?" Confucius is quoted as replying, "Yes!" Elaborating and confirming the point, he added that those who are intellectually and morally accomplished are temperate in their daily life, not overindulging themselves. They keep upright and unbiased in movement and stillness. They are temperate in joy and anger and hence do not pervert their intrinsic nature. It is all too natural that they should live long.

The Canon of Medicine further explores this line. It points out: "In caring for life, the wise must adapt themselves to the fluctuations of cold and heat in the four seasons, live peacefully and practise temperance in joy and anger, balance between yin and yang, strength and gentleness. Hence no outward evil can impair their health, and they enjoyed long lives.

Ancient Chinese thinkers advocated that the elderly think and study more. Guan Zi, a philosopher of the Warring States period, advised that "the elderly should always think." Xun Zi, a great Confucianist, argued that "learning should never cease"; that is, one is never too old to learn.

Yan Zhitui (531-c. 591), a scholar and man of letters of the Northern Qi Dynasty, declared that one should study tirelessly into old age, adding that the purpose of study is to "carry out the Dao for the benefit of the world" and cultivate oneself for improvement.

Ancient scholars on the art of healthy living advocated study and the use of the brain. Lü Shujian, a scholar in the Ming Dynasty, said: "One must often work hard with both mind and body. The harder one works with his mind, the more clever and resourceful one becomes; the harder one works with his body, the more healthy and robust one becomes."

Cao Huishan, a scholar in Qing times, wrote *Random Notes on Healthy Living* (*Lao Lao Heng Yan*), in which he advised people "not to give up studies just because of old age." He also indicated, "One cannot allow his mind to fall into disuse and must not let it turn into a piece of withered wood or dead ashes.... When it concentrates, it will not become fatigued in use." Therefore, a person who concentrates his mind on studies can be compared to a *qigong* practitioner who enters a quiescent mental state while thinking slightly of his *dantian* (a circular area below the navel). As an ancient couplet goes, "When sick, I do not fetch a physician; books nourish my health and life."

Practising *qigong* can prevent and cure diseases and prolong life. When one studies with absorbed attention, one dispels distracting thoughts just like a *qigong* master who is practising. So he gets the reward of *qigong* without practising it.

There were quite a number of "the wise" among ancient Chinese centenarians who made outstanding achievements in their later years. Sun Simiao, the "Master of Pharmacology" in the Tang Dynasty, wrote *The Thousand Golden Formulae* (*Qian Jin Yao Fang*) at the age of 70 and *Supplement to the Thousand Golden Formulae* (*Qian Jin Yi Fang*) at the age of 100. These works had a far-reaching influence on traditional Chinese medicine and even spread to Korea, Japan and other East Asian countries.

Another famous physician, Zhen Quan of Tang times, lived 103 years. He wrote *Acupuncture Prescriptions* (*Mai Jing Zhen Fang*) and some other important medical works. In his 103rd year, Tang Emperor Tai Zong visited him, asked him how he achieved such longevity and commended him.

Xie Qizuo, a native of Gaoyao in the Qing Dynasty, was still studying hard in his 90s. He took an imperial civil examination at the age of 95 and Emperor Qian Long appointed him a historian of the Imperial Academy to compile Chinese history. He was still alive at the age of 102.

Ni Tao, a native of Qiantang in the Qing Dynasty, devoted himself to studies all his life and continued to write books when he was more than 100 years old. His works include *Poring over the Book of Changes* (*Zhou Yi E Shu*) and *Record on One of the Six Arts* (*Liu Yi Zhi Yi Lu*).

Monk Xue Daoguang, a native of Jizushan of Shaanfu Prefecture in the Song Dynasty, had extensive learning and had once visited capital Changan to study. He wrote several books to explore Daoist *qigong* and its benefit to people's health and longevity. He died at the age of 114 after making much contribution to the Chinese art of healthy living.

The nine important formulae just discussed—following the principles of yin and yang, body-building exercises best-suited to one's condition, temperance in food and drink, a regular daily regimen, avoiding overexertion, keeping calm and cheerful, genetic strength, virtue and wisdom—present us with the secret of longevity of ancient Chinese centenarians.

It is clear that they did not owe their longevity to a single factor but to the combined results of these beneficial factors. Most centenarians emphasized one or two of them in accordance with their own circumstances, but they could not attain such longevity by paying attention only to one or two. In particular, the first six items are very important. Those centenarians who were highly distinguished paid special attention to the last two items. Moreover, family harmony and filial piety of children are especially beneficial for the longevity of family members. Therefore, a comprehensive plan for caring for life is an important principle in the traditional Chinese art of healthy living, as well as the secret of centenarians who distinguished themselves with their achievement.

Longevity in Contemporary Chinese Centenarians

In exploring longevity among ancient centenarians we aim at understanding its origins and in exploring longevity among contemporary centenarians, we aim at understanding its development. Only after understanding its origin and development can we get an overall view of longevity in China to provide reference for health care today.

According to statistics, the average life expectancy of a Chinese person was only 35 years in 1949 when the People's Republic of China was founded. It had risen to 69 by 1980 and exceeded 70 for urban dwellers.

In China's 1953 national census, 3,384 centenarians were found. In the third national census in 1982, 3,765 people of this age group were counted.

What is responsible for the longevity of today's centenarians?

The life-prolonging experiences of contemporary Chinese centenarians represent the development of an ancient tradition. Compared with ancient practices, these are of more relevance to people today.

As city-dwellers and rural people differ greatly in their daily habits, life styles, education, recreation and entertainment, as well as living environment, their life-prolonging practices will be dealt with separately.

Urban Centenarians

To explore the common laws of contemporary centenarians and at the same time reflect regional characteristics, four major cities are selected for analysis: Beijing in the north, Shanghai in the east, Guangzhou in the south and Chengdu in the west. Some centenarians with special traits or of typical significance in other cities are also dealt with below.

Beijing, the capital of China, had six centenarians in 1958 and 14 in 1981. In the third national census in 1982 the number of centenarians rose to 19, 16 women and 3 men, the oldest 104 years old. Thirteen of these centenarians were healthy and could attend to themselves in daily life. Some were able to do housework. Only five suffered from chronic diseases. Eleven of the centenarians lived in the city proper, seven in the suburbs and one on the outskirts.

Shanghai is a famous industrial city of China. Its oldest inhabitant in 1964 was 99 years old; it had six centenarians in 1973, 21 in 1979, and 23 in 1982 with the oldest 104 years old. Most centenarians lived downtown.

Guangzhou is a coastal city in south China. Now it has 22 centenarians, 19 women and 3 men, the oldest 110 years old. Seventeen of these centenarians care for themselves.

Chengdu, a major city in southwest China, is located in the centre of Sichuan Basin. In the 1982 national census it had 16 centenarians, 5 men and 11 women, the oldest 120 years old. Eleven lived in the city proper and five in the suburbs. Fourteen could care for themselves and do a little housework.

The four major cities had 80 centenarians at the third national census on July 1, 1982. It can be estimated there were nearly 100 centenarians in these cities in the early 1980s.

What is the secret of longevity of almost 100 city-dwelling centenarians? It can be summed up in the following aspects.

Regular Physical Labour; Body-Building Exercises

Most urban centenarians are in the habit of doing manual work. In their youth, female centenarians most did spinning and weaving, sewing, mending and laundry work; most male centenarians were peddlers, pedicab drivers and boatmen. Few did heavy physical labour. In old age they mainly do housework. None of them is an idler.

Grandma Chen Bingqing, 103 years old, is a Beijing inhabitant. She had earned her living in handicraft work in her youth. After the age of 80 she stays at home to care for her six grandchildren. She is busy from morning to night, neither inactive nor willing to be inactive. Although over 100, she remains hale and hearty. She has good vision, speaks clearly, moves about with ease and takes a stroll every day.

Chen Yanü, a 105-year-old Guangzhou woman, still goes shopping, washes clothes, cooks, and sews, threading needles without spectacles. When she visited her parental home in 1980, she rode in a long-distance bus for six hours and, eager to return home, walked so fast after getting off the bus that her great granddaughter-in-law could not keep up with her. This comes as a result of her doing manual work regularly.

Centenarian Grandpa Liu Shucheng, a gardener at Sichuan University in Chengdu, has tended flowers and plants for decades. He began gardening at the age of 18. Though retired, he still adds soil at the roots of flowers and plants, waters, prunes and applies manure on them every day, rain or sunshine. Thanks to long-term physical labour, the old man still has good vision and hearing, and remains healthy, robust and nimble. He looks like a man in his sixties.

All the above three urban centenarians do long-term manual work that is regular and temperate. This conforms to Sun Simiao's teaching, "The way of mental cultivation lies in frequent minor labour, but one should not be overfatigued or strain oneself beyond one's ability."

Centenarians who are intellectuals usually keep fit by doing physical exercises regularly. Ma Yinchu, a celebrated economist who suffered criticism and persecution in the "cultural revolution" because of his population control theory, lived through all these difficult years to be over 100 years old. He remained a sport lover all his life, and was fond of mountain climbing. At the age of 80 he climbed in high spirits to the Devil's Frown, the highest peak of the Fragrant Hills on the outskirts of Beijing.

When he was about 90 years old his legs were almost paralysed. Nevertheless, he consistently practised walking with crutches in the courtyard. Later, when his legs would no longer function, he supported his body with his hands on a square flower pot rack and walked forward laboriously, step by step. In order to assure that he had walked 6,000 to 7,000 paces every day, he used an ageold method of calculation. He put a given amount of broad beans in his left pocket and after walking over a certain distance, he shifted a broad bean from the left pocket into the right one. Only after all broad beans were thus shifted into the right pocket would he stop this exercise.

In 1972, Ma suffered from rectum cancer and had a surgery. After that he could not move about. Sitting in a wheelchair, this 91-year-old man wheeled himself repeatedly around his courtyard.

From youth to old age Professor Ma consistently took cold water baths. He first washed and rubbed his whole body with very hot water and then, soaking his towel in cold water, wrung it dry and rubbed himself until his body became red all over. Adhering to truth, Ma had a lifetime of frustrations, but he was able to live to the age of 100 because he kept doing physical exercises in harmony with the rhythm of his biological clock.

Elderly intellectuals are generally enthusiasts for *taijiquan*. Wu Tunan, a great *taijiquan* master, is also a scholar versatile in medical science, literature and archaeology and good at singing and playing music. His longevity is largely owing to his consistent practice of *taijiquan*. In 1984 at the age of 99 he won a prize at an international *taijiquan* exhibition in Wuhan.

In his early days Wu Tunan was very weak and suffered from multiple ailments, including pulmonary tuberculosis, infectious hepatitis, epilepsy and enlarged spleen. All the herbal decoctions he took could not help him. In his family he was believed to be doomed, but when he was nine years old his father took him to an imperial physician for treatment. Instead of prescribing medicinal herbs, the physician told the child to learn to practise traditional body-building exercises. So Wu went to learn from a *taijiquan* master, and showed his diligence and talent. It took him ten years to get rid of all his ailments, becoming for the first time healthy, strong and full of vitality. He graduated with an excellent academic record from the Metropolitan University, predecessor of Peking University.

To help more people improve their health, Wu Tunan wrote *Scientific Taijiquan* when he was only 23. Later he published *Studies of Taijiquan* and *The Science of Longevity*. He has done much work for the popularization and development of traditional Chinese body-building exercises.

Wu Tunan's wife used to be feeble in constitution. She practised *taijiquan* with Wu and was able to rid herself of all ailments. Ten years his junior, she is now in her 90s and still very healthy. She practises *taijiquan* and takes walks with Wu every day.

Many old city residents faithfully practise *qigong*, mostly dynamic-quiescent *qigong*. Peng Yutang, a doctor of traditional Chinese medicine, contracted pulmonary tuberculosis at the age of 48 from constant overwork as a silk-reeling worker. He spit blood and was bed-ridden. Later he practised "mind-cultivating dynamic-quiescent *qigong*" under the guidance of a famous master. He did it for three years and his lung trouble cleared without medical treatment. From then on he learned the art of traditional Chinese medicine from the master and became a physician. He continued to practise *qigong* after his recovery, enabling him to diagnose disease, write prescriptions and walk up to the third floor without panting when he was almost 100 years old.

He Xiqing, 104 years old, a native of Shanghai, holds that one should practise both meditation and active exercise. He became a Buddhist monk at 17 and learned from his master the art of meditation, which was a kind of quiet *qigong* exercise. He also learned martial arts in Tianjin in his early years. So he has practised quiet *qigong* and boxing all his life. Now, at the age of 104, he walks for two kilometres every morning from his home to Fuxing Park to practise boxing.

Brain Usage and Dedication to Work

Another prominent feature in the experiences of urban centenarian intellectuals is relentless use of the brain and dedication to work. As they plunge themselves heart and soul into their work and pin their hope on a distant goal, they remain calm, composed and optimistic even in the face of adversity.

Feng Gangbai, a centenarian painter of Guangzhou, has loved oil painting all his life. Art has produced a favourable influence on his character and has occupied his entire being. Feng said, "Painting makes me forget time and hardship and I attribute everything, including my life, to it." He has worked as an artist for over seven decades and experienced many difficulties and frustrations, but he can always remain calm and peaceful, ignoring honours or indignities. It is oil painting that gives him consolation and encouragement, becomes his spiritual pillar, tides him over many difficulties and enables him to live up to the present, brimming with vigour and confidence.

Su Juxian, 102 years old, is a calligrapher and member of the Shanghai Research Institute of Culture and History. He believes that calligraphy, like *qigong*, improves one's physical and mental health by bringing peace and harmony to the mind. He says, "Healthy living requires both quiet and active exercises. The meaning of active exercises is evident, but quietness is often mistaken to be passive sitting to rest the limbs and the brain. Actually, when one sits down to relax, he is troubled with various thoughts and cannot achieve quietness. True quietness can be found only in mental concentration, such as when one is absorbed in his work or study and forgets hunger or cold. When called, he forgets to respond; when disturbed, he becomes irritated. This can be considered as the state of quietness."

Sun Mofo, a participant of the 1911 Revolution, is now member of the Central Research Institute of Culture and History and Vice-President of the Chinese Society of Calligraphy and Painting of the Elderly. At the age of 104 he painted "Joy of Spring" on impulse when he attended a painting party to herald the arrival of spring in Beijing in 1985. Commenting on the relationship between calligraphy and good health, he said, "Calligraphy nourishes one's mind, nature, vital energy and life. When a calligrapher is using his brush, he naturally concentrates his mind wholly on his subject and puts away all other thoughts. He is deaf to wind or rain. Doesn't this have the same effect on one's health as *qigong*?"

These two calligraphers agree on the point that when one is doing wholeheartedly something he really likes to do, he can dispense with all other thoughts and achieve a mental state similar to that of *qigong* masters in deep meditation. He is therefore rewarded with good health and longevity.

Scientific studies show that man's cerebra begin to atrophy after the age of 40. But if one uses his brain regularly, it will atrophy more slowly, as shown in comparison between elderly people who study diligently and those who seldom use their brain. Using one's brain frequently can prevent senility.

Some urban centenarians also compose and recite poems and play chess. He Yongge, mother of the popular science writer Gao Shiqi, is a centenarian poet. Born in a family of scholars, she has loved writing poems and antithetical couplets since her youth. Inspired by poetry, she is cheerful and open-minded. When she was 100 years old and asked the secret of her longevity, she replied with a line of poetry, "Bullied by frost and snow, the flowering plum is all the more fragrant."

Her answer tells of a life of many frustrations. When her eldest daughter and favourite child died suddenly at the age of 23 she was so grieved she suffered a mental breakdown. Later, consoled by her family and drawing inspiration from poetry and books, she came to take her loss philosophically.

She encountered other tragedies. Eagerly looking forward to eldest son Gao Shiqi's return to China after completing his studies in the United States, her first sight was of him staggering as he walked, his neck stiff and his hands trembling. It turned out that while Gao studied in the United States, he accidentally contracted a virus in an experiment and suffered severe after-effects, all along concealing the circumstance from his mother. The reunion with her son brought her new sorrows.

But misfortunes sometimes continue and, in the winter of 1944 her husband, Gao Zanting, died of illness in Chongqing. But she was not to be beaten. Poetry consoled and inspired her to live on.

In the "cultural revolution" she suffered criticism and persecution like many other Chinese intellectuals of her generation, but she bore her misfortune with defiance and composure. That explains her artistic achievement and longevity.

Centenarian Xie Xiaxun, vice-chairman of the National Chess Association, has taken delight in playing chess all his life. From the age of six, he learned to play Chinese chess from his father. He won a Chinese chess championship in Shanghai in 1918 and later was hailed as "commander-in-chief of the national chess arena." In 1934 he was invited to visit Southeast Asia where he defeated the British international chess champion. He has been active in chess circles for over 90 years and written 29 books on chess. His daughter, Xie Bingchuan, explains why he has attained longevity, saying, "He recites poems, plays chess and his heart is serene and untroubled." He has inherited a precise secret of longevity, "quietness and serenety," from ancient Chinese centenarians.

Strict Daily Regimen

Urban residents mostly go to and from work on a schedule, a practice that helps many people cultivate good habits of work and rest according to a timetable. After retirement, most centenarians can also work and rest according to schedule. Some elderly people draw up a work-and-rest timetable for themselves, following it strictly.

Fan Heting, 102 years old, used to be an engineer in Shanghai. He retains good eyesight and hearing, and can still read and write. One of his secrets of longevity is strict observance of a work-and-rest timetable after retirement. He gets up at six each morning, has breakfast at seven and takes a walk in the park. He drinks milk at nine o'clock and has lunch at eleven. He takes a nap at one p.m., has some drinks such as malt-and-milk extract at three and supper at six, going to bed at nine. No matter how busy he is, he seldom disturbs this schedule.

Fan believes that "if one leads a regular life, he will always preserve his youth." If a machine operates on a regular pattern, it will be durable, and this applies to people. If one is too busy sometimes and too idle at others, doing whatever one likes, the regular pattern of human physiological activities will be undermined and components of the human body will be damaged. Engineer Fan takes good care of his body in the way he kept machines in good maintenance. Thanks to a regular life style, the major components of his body such as heart, brain, liver and lungs are normal, making him healthy and youthful.

Liao Fuhui of Guangzhou, 108 years old, has a more detailed work-and-rest timetable.

Four a.m.: Get up, wash face, drink tea and stretch limbs and waist.

Five thirty: Descend from the fourth floor, walk 1,000 metres to a tea house to take breakfast consisting of six *shaomai* (steamed meat dumplings with the dough gathered at the top) and a pot of fragrant tea.

Seven: Rest in bed for an hour.

Eight: Exercise to limber limbs and joints indoors and read books and newspapers for two hours.

Ten: Take light snack (mix a beaten egg into a glass of milk), do limbering-up exercises and self-massage.

Twelve noon: Take lunch, a small bowl of rice and simple dishes. (He is not particular about food, but he loves fish.)

Twelve-thirty p.m.: Take a nap for an hour.

One thirty: Descend from the fourth floor and go to tea house to drink tea, take light refreshments and chat with others.

Four-thirty: Indoor activity. Watch a game of chess or play chess with great grandson, chat with others and read pictorials.

Six: Take supper, a small bowl of rice and a small bowl of soup.

Seven: Watch TV.

Ten: Light snack, a small bowl of sugar water or one *liang* (fifty grams) of noodles.

Ten-thirty: Go to bed.

Liao used to be a merchant travelling between Hong-kong, Singapore and Malaysia. After the founding of People's Republic of China he settled down in Guangzhou and has followed this regimen throughout over three decades. Now, he has a pair of bright, piercing eyes, speaks in a loud, clear voice and walks with vigorous strides. He neither breathes hard nor rests when going upstairs. He walks several *li* (half a kilometre) without feeling tired and brims with zest for life.

Rational Diet; Avoid Smoking and Alcohol

Urban centenarians neither indulge in fine food nor pay too much attention to nutrition. They never overeat, and seldom smoke or drink alcohol.

Beijing residents have wheat flour as staple food, while people in Shanghai, Guangzhou and Chengdu mostly eat rice. Non-staple foods consist mainly of fresh vegetables. In Beijing there are fewer vegetables in winter while Shanghai, Guangzhou and Chengdu have fresh vegetables throughout the seasons. Chengdu is endowed with most favourable conditions for growing vegetables. It has a rich variety of vegetables of good quality and low price. Centenarians, in general, eat meat, but only in limited amounts, though some in Chengdu have a fairly good appetite for meat.

In arranging three daily meals, most elderly people consume milk and egg at breakfast; meat, vegetables, rice or food made of wheat flour at lunch, and a little simple food at supper. Their food contains much protein, a limited amount of animal fat and some sugar and vitamins. The metabolic process in the elderly is mainly involved in decomposition, requiring fairly abundant proteins for compensation. Consequently, the elderly ought to eat food abundant in protein, such as milk, eggs, fish and beans.

Elderly people also require meat in their diets. Lean meat contains mainly protein and fat meat has a lot of fat, which is needed to some degree because vitamins A, D, K and E cannot dissolve and be absorbed without fat. Vitamins A and E have multiple functions of combatting cancer and prolonging life. Vitamin D can prevent elderly people from calcium deficiencies and protect them from osteoporosis and fractures. Vitamin K prevents rupture of blood vessels and haemorrhage. If one avoids or eats too little animal fat, it will lead to deficiencies in the above-mentioned vitamins. Moreover, animal blood and fat contain high density lipoprotein that can prevent cholesterol from causing arteriosclerosis and obviate coronary heart disease and hypertension.

Both 120-year-old Zheng Hongxin of Chengdu and 102-year-old Zhou Kun of Beijing like to eat meat, fat or lean, and neither suffers from hypertension or coronary heart disease. Thus it is possible to benefit from fat while eliminating its harm.

Elderly people, with their comparatively low rates of metabolism, do a limited amount of physical activity, hence they need consume only small quantities of heat unit foods. Thus, they should eat limited amounts of rice and wheat flour which produce a large quantity of heat. Urban brain workers and others whose physical activities are limited should also eat little sugar.

Centenarian Liao Fuhui of Guangzhou eats less than one *liang* of rice at a meal, about four *liang* (120 grams) a day. Chen Bingqing, a 103-year-old woman, says, "One should not eat a lot of food. Sixty percent of full is enough." This conforms to the ancient theory that one who eats little lives long.

In one experiment related to food quantities, when white mice with unrestricted access to food died, most of the mice for whom food quantities were limited survived. Other scientists exploring the effects of nutrition on life span and health found that mice in a food-restricted group had longer life spans than those of the non-restricted group; fewer suffered from nephritis and cancer, and diseases occurred later in life among them.

Experiments have also shown that restricting one's food intake during the early teens will be helpful in prolonging life. Ultimately, restrictions on food quantities in old age tend to reduce or eliminate effects of damage caused by previous overeating. Some scientists estimate from experiments on animals that one can prolong one's life by 40 years if one limits his or her food consumption.

Centenarians in different regions have different habits in food and drink, some of which are beneficial. For instance, centenarians in Beijing like to eat garlic, while those in Guangzhou and Shanghai like to eat fish and those in Chengdu like to eat chilli and pickles.

Garlic helps prevent and cure arteriosclerosis, reduce blood-fat and prevent myocardial infarction among the middle-aged and old people. It is effective in reducing fat and combatting coagulation, helping prevent cerebral thrombosis. Garlic can also stimulate the pituitary to control the function of some endocrine glands and adjust absorption of fat and sugar. Consequently, it is helpful for combatting obesity and diabetes.

Scientists have also discovered that garlic has some effect against cancer. It can kill bacteria and prevent enteritis and pneumonia. Therefore, centenarians fond of eating garlic seldom suffer from the above-mentioned diseases. Sun Ping of Wuqiang County in Hebei Province is now 101 years old. She likes to eat garlic and has no other preference in food. She was afflicted with severe stomach trouble at the age of 40. Later she ate one or two garlics every day for over six decades. Since then she has never had stomach pains. Moreover, medical checkups show that nothing is wrong with her heart, lungs, liver or spleen.

Fish is a favourite dish for almost everybody. Fish contain much protein and little fat and the meat is easy to digest, very suitable for elderly people. Incidence of heart disease ranks lowest in China among the fishermen of Zhoushan Islands. Centenarians in Shanghai and Guangzhou eat large amounts of fish, resulting in good cardiovascular conditions.

Chengdu residents like to eat chilli and pickles. These two kinds of food can help reduce blood-fat, dissolve and digest fat and prevent cardiovascular diseases. Chilli can also promote secretion of digestive juices and peristalses of the stomach and intestines to aid digestion. Chilli is packed with vitamin C. Half a kilogram of red pepper contains one gram of vitamin C and also provitamin A. Vitamin C can prevent arteriosclerosis, improve body resistance and prevent cancer. Provitamin A can be turned into vitamin A which assists in preventing cancer and combatting senility.

Some ancient Daoist priests believed that eating chilli can prolong human life. In *Compendium of Ancient and Modern Medical Literature (Gu Jin Yi Tong Da Quan)*, a comprehensive medical book edited by the Ming scholar Xu Chunfu, it is recorded that elderly people on Qingcheng Mountain who ate chilli over a long time achieved longevity.

Pickles are prepared by soaking chilli, turnips and other vegetables in light salt water, preserving vitamin C in the vegetables. Tasting slightly sour, pickles whet the appetite and help break down fat and grease. Pickles, sometimes stir-fried with meat, taste delicious and can prevent unfavourable side effects caused by excessive fat. Chengdu centenarians who are fond of eating meat, in general, do not have high levels of cholesterol.

Aside from their special tastes, centenarians in Beijing, Shanghai, Guangzhou and Chengdu all have one preference in common—drinking tea. Grandma Zhang nee Men, 105 years old, as well as Wang Changshun and Li Yukang, both 101 years old, all drink tea every day. More than half of the Shanghai centenarians have been fond of drinking tea since their youth. Grandma Zhang Dianxiu, 104 years old, always drinks a cup of black tea after getting up, the first thing she does every day. Nearly all Chengdu centenarians like to drink jasmine tea.

Now scientists have discovered that drinking tea can prevent cancer and combat diabetes. Zhejiang Medical University has discovered that pigments in tea leaves can prevent vascular sclerosis. In the 120 cases when physicians at the hospital affiliated with the university treated atherosclerosis with pigment extracted from tea leaves, the effective rate reached 82 percent.

Recent studies have shown that the tannic acid of tea leaves can inhibit the birth of ester peroxidate that leads to the senility of cells. Experiments have shown that the anti-senility effects of tea leaves are 19 times higher than those of vitamin E.

One in every four elderly people in Guangzhou often drink the "Guangzhou sugar water." Among its ingredients, the refined cane sugar contains multiple trace elements necessary for the human body. Beans contain abundant plant protein. Hyacinth beans strengthen the spleen and are diuretic. Red beans and green beans are antipyretic. Edible seaweeds are called "vegetables of longevity." They contain mutiple minerals and vitamins and the rich iodine content can reduce storage of fat in the body and prevent hyperlipemia, coronary heart disease and hypertension.

Edible seaweeds also exert a curative effect on chronic bronchitis, and dried bean milk cream rolls contain very high protein content. One hundred gram of such rolls contain 50.5 grams of protein and 598 milligrams of iodine. Guangzhou sugar water, therefore, has a complete nutritive range as a beneficial health drink for the elderly in tropical and sub-tropical regions.

A considerable number of centenarians establish the habit of more but smaller meals each day. For instance, six out of ten elderly people in Guangzhou take five to six meals a day, eating up to one *liang* (50 grams) of grain at each meal. This is an inherited experience in longevity from ancient Chinese centenarians of eating frequent small meals in place of large meals.

In a study of 1,400 people between 60 and 64 who ingested normal amounts of calories, 668 ate one or two meals a day and one in three suffered from cardiovascular diseases. Another 156 of these people divided the same amount of food into five meals a day and only one in six suffered from cardiovascular disease. This confirms that eating less in more meals is a beneficial habit for the elderly.

Eight of ten urban centenarians neither smoke nor drink alcoholic beverages. Those who smoke consume less than five cigarettes a day, and those who drink consume only small amounts of liquor, about one *liang* a day. None drink excessively.

Drinking a small amount of liquor is beneficial to elderly people. It facilitates digestion and promotes blood circulation. Studies show that drinking a small amount of fruit wine can reduce likelihood of heart diseases.

Prompt Treatment; Proper Rest and Nourishment

China's cities have better medical facilities and more skilled physicians than rural areas. People there also have a fuller and broader knowledge of health care.

In general, timely diagnosis and treatment for diseases is more readily available in urban areas, and emergency rescue systems are more effective. This helps reduce the mortality rate, one reason the average life expectancy of city residents exceeds 70, higher than that of rural dwellers.

Grandma Sun Wanfang, 102 years old, of Huangpu district in Shanghai, was saved by prompt emergency treatment when she suffered from severe stomach trouble and several massive haemorrhages in her thirties. After recovering, Grandma Sun developed physical health by taking smaller but more meals, coupled with medicines. Since then she has had no stomach trouble and remains healthy at the age of more than 100.

Of course, it is of little value for one to rely only on good medical facilities if knowledge of health care is lacking and one fails to build health through proper rest and nutrition. Centenarian Guo Yangyuan used to suffer from many diseases such as hypertension, migraine, arthritis and neurasthenia, which were little helped by medicines. After retiring at the age of 70 he read many books on the art of healthy living and learned to do self-massage. Months after, his blood pressure dropped from 190/120 (mm Hg) to 170/100 (mm Hg), his dizziness ceased, his appetite returned, he slept better and his walk was more springy. These initial effects gave him the confidence to continue. From extensive reading and personal experience, he worked out a set of massage best fitted to himself. A year later he stopped taking medicines and his diverse diseases gradually vanished.

Twenty years later, however, he was afflicted with cancer twice, one at the age of 92 and again when he was 94. He improved after timely diagnosis and treatment, but after a second operation for bladder cancer, he was bed-ridden for two months from excessive bleeding. Once his health improved, he started again to massage himself and follow a strict daily regimen. He developed a schedule of balanced nutrition for himself after consulting a number of books on health care:

Six a.m.: A soft-boiled egg, a small bowl of porridge, and a slice of steamed roll with salted vegetables or pickles, sesame paste or fermented bean curd.

Ten-thirty a.m.: A bowl of milk or vegetable soup, occasionally with an egg added.

Twelve noon: A few spoonfuls of soup, then one *liang* of rice and a dish of vegetable (its variety changing from time to time) stir-fried with lean pork or a dish of fish.

Six p.m.: One *liang* of steamed roll or pancake, one *liang* of rice or cornmeal porridge and a dish of bean products or fresh vegetables. Occasionally a small amount of beer or Shaoxing rice wine. Fruit after supper.

Apart from taking meals according to the schedule, Grandpa Guo Yangyuan also follows a regimen in his daily life: Get up at five every day. Massage himself before washing face. Take an outdoor stroll for half an hour. After breakfast listen to a news broadcast and take a walk in the park at eight. After snack at ten-thirty rest for half an hour, then read books and practise calligraphy. After lunch do housework, then read newspapers and take a nap. Walk outdoors at three p.m. and go shopping. Do housework. After supper rest for half an hour, read popular science periodicals and watch TV. At nine p.m. go to bed and massage himself for half an hour before falling asleep.

Grandpa Guo Yangyuan paid attention to proper rest and nutrition and cooperated closely with physicians in treatment to, at long last, defeat cancer. At the age of 100, he still moves about with ease, speaks clearly and remains as lively in thinking and memory as in earlier years.

Environment and Hygiene

Cities are densely populated with heavy traffic and factory concentrations, causing comparatively severe environmental pollution. These are damaging to good health and longevity. Many older residents tend flowers and plants to beautify the environment, purify the air and help them with physical exercise.

Most Chengdu centenarians make a hobby of growing and cherishing flowers. They have flowers and plants throughout their homes. With cottonrose hibiscus flowers dominant in streets and lanes, Chengdu used to be known as "City of the Cottonrose

Hibiscus." They have been replaced by exotic flowers and plants introduced in recent years. Flowers not only adorn the city and purify the air but can also brighten up the mind of the growers.

Veteran Red Army man Ding Shixiong, 103 years old, has been spending all his time in his small garden since his retirement. There he has planted a rich variety of flowers: primrose and magnolia in spring; garden balsam and canna in summer; marigold and orange osmanthus in autumn and camellia and red plum in winter. He also has such precious plants as kafir lily, peony, orchid cactus and aglais. Especially eye-catching is his kumquat plant laden with fruit. His flowers, indeed, can rival those in the city's Qingyang-gong Temple.

Ding has beautified the environment with his hands and has reduced air and noise pollution. He remains radiant with vitality and his face glows with health at the age of 103.

Flowers are known as "natural physicians." The aroma of geraniums (*Pelargonium hortorum*) has a tranquilizing effect, dissipating fatigue and inducing sleep. Two pots of geraniums in the bedroom will help one fall asleep quickly. The fragrance of jasmine can regulate the circulation of *qi*, making people relaxed and cheerful. The delicate aroma of lotus flower and rugosa rose can prevent attacks of coronary heart disease. The scent of Cape jasmine benefits liver and gall and helps prevent and cure hepatitis and cholecystitis, and the fragrance of lilac can purify the air and kill bacteria. Experiments show that its bacteria-killing capacity is six times as powerful as carbolic acid. A perfume bag of dried lilac blossoms hung in a room or on one's body can help prevent pulmonary tuberculosis and chronic gastro-enteritis, and the rich scent of cordate telosma repels mosquitoes so people can enjoy summer life without being harrassed. That scent can also help prevent malaria.

Many flowers can also be used as medicine. For instance, honeysuckle is antipyretic and alleviates inflammation, the self-heal blossom (*Prunella vulgaris*) can improve vision and lower blood pressure and the aroma of the hyacinth bean flower whets the appetite. In ancient times a folk saying held that if one eats chrysanthemums over a long time, he can attain longevity.

It is interesting that flowers can announce the hours: Morning glory blossoms at four a.m., the break of day. Mei Lanfang, a great master of Beijing opera, loved morning glory mostly because the flower could prompt him to get up early to practise singing and acrobatic skills. Herbaceous peony blooms in a broad smile at seven a.m., lotus flowers spread their petals at nine and magnolia is in full bloom at ten.

Sweet-scented flowers and plants broaden people's vision and ease their mind. Therefore, as somebody once said, "Whoever loves flowers lives long."

Grandma Pei nee Fu of Taiyuan, 103 years old, loves flowers as much as life. North China is covered with ice and snow in winter and hardly a green leaf can be found, but Grandma Pei's courtyard brims with the charms of spring. She began growing flowers in her thirties after her husband's death, even when she did laundry for others to earn a living and support her three children. It is flowers that have given her consolation, happiness, and courage to survive hardships.

She has been tending flowers for the past seven decades. As soon as she hears of a beautiful flower somewhere, she will go great distances to see or acquire it. When she was 103 years old, she carried a pot of flowers home from about three kilometres away. With her diligent hands she has preserved spring in her courtyard and her youth as well. Now she is still nimble, dexterous and quick in her movements just as a young woman.

All Chinese city centenarians have good hygienic habits. They consistently rinse mouths; brush teeth and frequently cut their fingernails; change their linen, quilts and bed sheets, and wash their feet before bed-time each day. Most sweep their courtyards and keep their rooms clean and tidy. Grandma Tang Shengyun of Chengdu, 101 years old, sweeps her courtyard three times a day and keeps her room bright and clean without a speck of dust. Grandma Li Ying of Guangzhou, 107 years old, is known as "Clean Grandma" in the neighbourhood. She takes a sponge bath with warm water three times a day, lasting 40 minutes each time, the good habit established through perseverance. Centenarians mostly have good hygienic habits and therefore seldom fall ill.

Rural Centenarians

What is the key to the longevity of centenarians in rural China that has its own characteristics and advantages? According to the survey and analysis of Chinese medical scientists on longevity, centenarians in the rural areas of Xinjiang, Sichuan, Guangxi and Guangdong have a number of characteristics in common, ranging from a quiet environment and fresh air to a willingness to help others.

Quiet Environment and Fresh Air

In China's vast countryside many places have fresh air and beautiful environments where hills, though not high, are green throughout the seasons and streams, though not deep, are fresh and clear. In particular, a zone of longevity can be identified from the northwest through the southwest to the south. Bansheng Township of Du'an County in Guangxi is especially noted as a home of longevity in China with up to 23 centenarians among its 20,000 inhabitants.

Bansheng Township is situated in mountains ranging from 1,000 to 1,500 metres above sea level. Woods cover the hills with luxuriant foliage for a lush, green beauty in all seasons. Most centenarians live half way up the mountain or higher, and only a few live on the lower slopes. Although it is in the sub-tropical zone, the climate is mild and pleasant in the mountains. According to meteorological records in 1959, the highest temperature that year was 36.5°C and the lowest temperature 4°C, with a mean temperature in June of 26.2°C. The average annual temperature was 17.8 °C with a total precipitation of 1,455 millimetres. Precipitation was 381.4 millimetres in June and 1.1 in October, with fairly high precipitation in June-August period cooling summer heat.

Houses on the mountains are multi-level buildings made of bamboo and wood with good ventilation.

People live upstairs to avoid ground-level humidity. Many fruit and other trees and small vegetable gardens are laid out around the houses. The environment is quiet, secluded, without air or noise pollution. Trees provide verdant shade and streams are always clear.

Yangcun Village on the Ganjiang River and on the outskirts of Nanchang, the capital of Jiangxi Province, is one of the world's six best villages for longevity today. The village has over 40 households with 335 people, 106 of whom are above sixty. Eight villagers are in their nineties. The average life expectancy of the villagers is nearly 80.

The beautiful scenery of the village is thick with more than 20,000 trees of different varieties, averaging 70 trees per resident. All the farm houses nestle in the midst of trees and bamboo.

On the Ganjiang River, Yangcun Village has plenty of delicious fish and shrimps and fresh vegetables throughout the seasons and a great variety of fruits and melons. Villagers eat fresh, nourishing vegetables all around the year.

The village is not naturally endowed with this beautiful environment but relies entirely on afforestation. Some 10,000 shade trees and vast expanses of fruit trees have all been planted by the villagers themselves.

Such broad expanses of green plants have a favourable influence on climate. Although summer climate in Nanchang is intolerably hot, Yangcun Village remains cool and refreshing. Man cannot live without oxygen and green plants serve as oxygen makers. One hectare of broad-leaf forests can release 730 kilograms of oxygen, absorb 1,000 kilograms of carbon dioxide and purify 1,800 cubic metres of air.

Many plants secrete substances that kill bacteria. For instance, pines can release pungent oxygen with very high bactericidal power. Eucalyptus, lemon and camphor trees, birches and poplars can secrete a large amount of aromatic bacteriocidin. Wherever afforestation has been well carried out, viruses and bacteria in the air are noticeably reduced. People living in such an environment are less susceptible to diseases. Green plants can also absorb sulfur dioxide and other harmful gases. Pine forests can absorb 29 milligrams of sulfur dioxide in a cubic metre of air each day. A hectare of willows can absorb 10 kilograms of sulfur dioxide every month during the growing season.

Some scientists believe that 80 percent of cancer is caused by air pollution. Most cases of senile tracheitis and asthma are caused by sulfur dioxide gas plus the stimulus of cold air. Afforestation can greatly reduce these diseases detrimental to elderly people. Green plants can also absorb dust and alleviate noise pollution. The leaf surface of the plants mostly has fine down and can secrete viscous juice so it can absorb dust in the air. Tree-thick zones contain 50 percent less dust than non-forest zones.

Green plants can regulate the nervous system, cerebral cortex and retina tissue, steady pulses, stabilize blood pressure and improve vision. Places with green tree shade have plenty of negative ions in the air. Investigations show many times more air negative ions in forests than in central cities. Inhaling such negative ions can refresh the brain and invigorate the spirit. Negative ion is also called "air vitamin" and "longevity element in the air." It has the function of tranquilizing the mind, alleviating pain, relieving cough and spasms and facilitating urination. It also helps prevent and cure senile diseases such as hypertension, chronic tracheitis and bronchial asthma. Elderly people can stroll and practise *taijiquan* in the woods to fight chronic ailments. It is now called "forest therapy."

The richly endowed natural conditions of rural areas, coupled with afforestation, can create a living environment superior to that of cities and beneficial to health and longevity.

Plain Living; Energetic Life

Living centenarians in China's countryside mostly have experienced decades of hardship. They worked hard all year long to earn livelihoods.

Sichuan Province has 330 rural centenarians. With the exception of one person, all used to be poor peasants, most having endured hardships from their early days. Of about 300 centenarians, 36 were forced to be child brides. Precisely because their families were poor, they had to earn their livings by hard work. Physical labour has given them strong physique and the habit of constantly exercising the body. Although they are 100 years old now, they still continue to work, accepting the adage that "running water is never stale and a door-hinge never gets worm-eaten." Many years of labour has strengthened their tendons and bones and they do not grow decrepit in old age.

Eight out of ten rural centenarians are women, who spin and weave, raise pigs, cook, grow vegetables and water the fields. Such work does not cause overfatigue but keeps the body's vitality.

Grandma Tang Shuhua became a child bride at the age of nine. She first cut grass and firewood, and when a little older did farm work in the fields. Now 124 years old, she is still able to go uphill with a walking stick to gather firewood and wild vegetables.

Shu Junhe, the oldest living centenarian in Hunan Province, is also a peasant who has endured hardship. Born of a poor family, he has worked as hired farm worker, stonemason, carpenter and bricklayer. Decades of physical labour has made him strong and robust. In his youth he could carry a 150-kilogram stone grinder on shoulder poles and still walk with a vigorous step. Now 112 years old, he still has a steady gait and can carry a load of some 30 kilograms on shoulder poles. Though his sons and grandsons advise him to enjoy his old age in leisure, he cannot stay idle for even a day. He often goes uphill to gather firewood or waters vegetables in the fields. When some visitors come from far away, he will wade barefoot in a river to catch fish and shrimps to offer guests a warm welcome.

Li Guangzhen, 105 years old and a native of Naxi County in Sichuan Province, became a child bride at the age of seven and earned her living for nearly a century spinning yarn and weaving hemp cloth. She is still able to do housework.

Grandma Ran, 109 years old, a peasant of Yishan County in Guangxi, was a deputy to the Fifth National People's Congress. She has done manual labour since childhood. Year in and year out, this has been a habit, one that makes her feel ill at ease if she stops working for a single day. She can still sow, manure, earth up crops and weed fields.

Grandma Chen nee Tian, 121 years old, lives in a high,

cold mountainous area in Guizhou Province. At three she lost her mother and the year after the next her father died. At eight she left the famine-stricken village with her paternal aunt, roaming and begging. At 16 she earned a living as a seasonal farm hand. Although she has eaten plain and simple food most of her life, hardship has built her strong body. Now she can still carry 10 kilograms of wild medicinal herbs on her back on medical visits to villages 15 kilometres away. She also raises pigs and chickens. She remains sober-minded and nimble and has good vision, though she is somewhat hard of hearing.

There are also a number of centenarians who have learned martial arts and practised boxing in their off hours to strengthen their physiques.

Centenarian Yang Weiyuan in a village on Yangquan's outskirts in Shanxi Province was born to a very poor family. At the age of nine he carried vegetables on shoulder poles to sell at the fair. Frequent burdens such as this bend his spine and he developed into a humpbacked boy by the age of 12, earning the name "Humpbacked Vegetable Boy." Later he heard that martial arts can both strengthen one's body and help in self-defence. So he became a disciple of a boxing master in his village and practised boxing mornings and evenings under the master's guidance. In three or four years his humpback had straightened. From then on he practised boxing and wielded a cudgel or other weapon with dedication.

He was chosen as martial arts referee for the provincial sports meet in 1958 and more than 40 young lads are now learning martial arts from him. Although 100 years old, he is still strong and robust, walks with a steady gait and is nimble in movement. He has bright piercing eyes and his youthful countenance is in delightful contrast to his white hair.

Grandma Liu Guoqing, 108 years old, lives in Tea Garden Ravine, Sanyi Township, Shizhu Tujia Autonomous County, Sichuan Province. She can perform "Bird and Animal Boxing of Emei" and can carry two buckets of water (37 kilograms) over a distance of three hundred metres. She can also lift a 34-kilogram bench effortlessly with three fingers and hold a bucket of water weighing 18.5 kilograms in her teeth. She is tall and has black, glossy hair and a ruddy complexion. With her guidance, five of her six family members are skilled at martial arts and have set up a martial arts school.

Liu Guoqing was born to a poor peasant family in the shadow of Emei Mountain and learned "Bird and Animal Boxing of Emei." Sold because of poverty at the age of seven to an acrobatic troupe from Jiangsu Province, she earned her living as a performer. She also learned jujitsu, rope dancing and the use of various weapons. Later she left the acrobatic troupe to marry a young martial arts master named Peng. Settling in the countryside, she has continued practising martial arts for decades. Under her influence her son, grandson and great grandson all loved boxing and martial arts so that the Pengs have become a family known far and near for their martial arts skills.

Eating What Is Available; Whole Grains as the Staple

Rural centenarians, in general, are not particular about their selection of food and drink, eating whatever is at hand. And they eat mostly whole grain cereals rather than polished rice and wheat flour as their staple food. In the north they eat mainly maize, millet and beans. In the south they eat sweet potatoes in addition to maize and beans. They all eat more fresh vegetables than city residents, but southerners eat more than northerners.

Compared with polished rice and wheat flour, maize and millet are higher in nutritional value, containing twice as much cellulose needed by elderly people and larger amounts of trace elements and vitamins. Beans, soybeans in particular, contain the largest amount of protein among food grains and are suited to needs of the elderly.

Sweet potato is very widespread in the rural areas. It almost becomes staple food in Sichuan Province with the exception of mountainous areas in western Sichuan. Villagers usually eat sweet potato at least six months each year. It contains more protein, vitamin C and carotene than polished rice or wheat flour. It also contains mucin, which can reduce occurrence of atherosclerosis and obesity. Some scientists believe it can prevent atrophy of connective tissues in the liver and stomach and other diseases of connective tissues, and maintain the lubrication of digestive and respiratory tracts, joints and serous membranes. Cellulose in sweet potatoes can also facilitate bowel movement. Consequently, sweet potato is beneficial for old people, helping them against hypertension, coronary heart disease, arteriosclerosis, constipation and obesity.

Recently, scientists have extracted from sweet potatoes a chemical substance called DHEA (dehydroepiandrosterone). It is a steroid similar to adrenalin. When injected with DHEA, white mice raised for the culture of cancerous cells no longer suffered from colon and mammary cancers and survived for 36 months. On the other hand, those white mice without DHEA injection had only a life expectancy of 24 months. Evidently, this chemical substance can prolong the life span of white mice by one third. Likewise, people who eat sweet potato can also prolong their lives.

Rural centenarians eat whole grain cereals as their main staple food, a practice that conforms to old people's physiological conditions. In particular, cellulose contained in whole grain cereals is necessary for the elderly. It can prevent habitual constipation and cancer in intestines.

As rural centenarians eat plenty of vegetables and whole grain cereals and drink hard water (containing trace elements such as calcium and magnesia), they seldom suffer from heart and brain vascular diseases. The blood pressure of 127-year-old Grandma Mengama of Guangxi measures 140/86 (mm Hg), her cardiac sounds are powerful and her rhythm regular. Her cardiovascular conditions are as good as those of a healthy person in his fifties. The soil of areas such as Xinjiang also contains zinc and manganese, trace elements beneficial to cardiac blood vessels. Incidences of hypertension and coronary heart disease are therefore relatively low there.

Rural centenarians generally have good appetites and eat large amounts of food. So do most of the 300 rural centenarians in Sichuan. Grandpa Yuan Kaixing of Pingchang County, 106 years old, now consumes half a catty (250 grams) of meat, two *liang* (50 grams) of liquor and a catty of cooked rice every day. Grandma

Liu Guoqing of Shizhu County, 108 years old, eats a catty of cooked rice at a meal. Consumption for these people is consistent with their physical activities and they tend to have little surplus nourishments stored in the body to cause harm. So people who mainly do mental work can live long if they eat little, while those who mainly do manual work can maintain good health and prolong their lives even if they eat plenty. This does not mean they can overeat, however.

A considerable number of rural centenarians are fond of eating meat in their late years; very few are true vegetarians. Only 12 of the 300 centenarians in Sichuan Province have been vegetarians throughout their lives. Others generally like to eat meat, some even eat a catty of pork at a meal. Zhou Hongfu, a peasant of Zhejiang Province, drank almost half a catty of liquor and ate nearly a kilogram of pork in celebration of his 80th birthday. Grandpa Zheng Zhaohe, 103 years old, of Tongbai mountainous area in Hubei Province, was also fond of eating meat. On his 103rd birthday the old couple (his wife was 106 years old) ate a two-kilogram chicken in one meal.

We must understand that these old people like to eat meat because it is not often available and especially because they were poor and seldom ate meat in their youth. So when they occasionally eat pork at a meal, they eat plenty. An oldster who eats several catties of meat at a meal without any ailment or trouble confirms that he has good digestion, strong stomach and physique. But such practice of overeating at a meal is very detrimental to the elderly's health and must not be encouraged.

Why do few rural centenarians suffer from coronary

heart disease and arteriosclerosis even though they like to eat meat? Preference for meat does not mean eating meat every day. On ordinary days most of them eat simple, plain food and few eat meat once a week. Of course, a few can eat one or two *liang* of meat every day and still be healthy.

Surveys and studies have shown that when elderly people above 60 eat moderate amount of meat, this will not cause arteriosclerosis or coronary heart disease. A survey of 88 centenarians in Hubei Province has shown that 34 percent suffered from starvation in childhood and in the prime of their lives. Starvation in this period helped them through the period of high incidence of coronary arteriosclerosis. Middle age is the key period in the formation of coronary arteriosclerosis, which can therefore be prevented by dieting and eating little meat in this period.

Centenarians now alive in China's countryside were often underfed and seldom ate meat before their sixties and seventies because of younger lives of misery and hardship. Rural elderly people have many physical chores to attend to, consuming energy and reducing the harm of meat. Unlike urban people, they need not be "as wary of fat meat as of a tiger." Moreover, the Chinese have the habit of cooking meat with vegetables. Vitamin C and cellulose in vegetables help in digesting meat and prevent the deposit of too much cholesterol in the body. The fat in meat is beneficial to the absorption of fat-soluble vitamins.

Rural elderly people generally eat food with little salt because many people live in mountainous areas with poor transportation and salt is as costly as gold. Bama County, a home of longevity in Guangxi, lacks salt so people there eat food with little or no salt and hypertension is seldom found among them. Salt promotes contraction of blood vessels, which increases the burden on the heart and causes hypertension. So elderly people should restrict their salt intake to about five grams each day.

Xinjiang has 865 centenarians, the largest concentration in China. There are two major characteristics in their diet: fondness for melons and fruit and the drinking of sour milk.

Xinjiang is nationally famous for its grapes and Hami melons. Grandpa Abdulla's family lives in Garden Village of Grape Township in Turpan County. Abdulla, 117 years old, lives in a family with five generations of more than 200 members under one roof. His eldest son is 96 years old and his youngest son in his sixties. People call the Abdullas the "family of longevity." The key to their longevity lies in "eating melons and fruits," as each person eats some 250 kilograms a year. Grapes here were recorded more than 2,000 years ago in *Shen Nong's Materia Medica* (*Shen Nong Ben Cao Jing*) for their function in strengthening tendons and bones and prolonging life.

Grandma Song Jinniang in Ruisui Township, Hualian County in Taiwan, was born on January 1, 1874. She is now the oldest person in Taiwan, Apart from being optimistic and fond of physical exercises, she mainly likes to eat betel nuts. Chinese in the south have eaten betel nuts since ancient times. People south of the Five Ridges (the area covering Guangdong and Guangxi) substitute betel nuts for tea, believing they can resist evil vapours rising from marshes. Traditional Chinese medical theory holds that betel nuts can regulate the flow of vital energy, remove obstructions, aid digestion and kill parasites.

In Yengisar County, Xinjiang, there is a family that has five centenarians. One of them, Turdi Salay, 136 years old, is China's oldest living person. Drinking sour milk over a long time is what this family sees as responsible for the longevity of its members. Sour milk contains natural antibacterial substances and can inhibit cancer. In an experiment with cancerous mice, one group was fed sour milk and the other group received other food without sour milk. The cancer in the first group of mice was inhibited and growth of cancerous cells reduced 30 to 35 percent.

Some centenarians, particularly those in Sichuan Province, are especially fond of eating sugar. Centenarians in other regions also eat a great deal of sugar, mainly the brown sugar which is better than refined white sugar or crystal sugar for its multiple trace elements and vitamins.

Rural residents mainly do manual work which consumes large quantities of heat. So their food should differ from that of city residents mainly engaged in mental work.

There are different views on the question of elderly people eating sugar. Some scientists believe that with the exception of tooth decay, almost no evidence has been found to support the view that eating sugar is unfavourable to health. But it is best neither to emphasize abstaining from sugar nor to consume too much. And it is better for diabetics and overweight persons to take care with sugar.

Most rural centenarians eat three meals a day and some only two, but most have developed the good habit of eating a light supper. In one interesting experiment two groups of people take only one meal with each group's food identical each day. One group eats at seven a.m. and the other group eats at five-thirty p.m. Those eating in the morning gradually lose weight while evening eaters steadily gain weight. Evidently, adequate food in the morning meets energy needs for the day's work without making people fat. It is not good for one to overeat in the evening, because insulin in the blood increases to its peak at dusk and blood sugar is turned into fat and stored beneath the abdominal wall. When continued over a long period this results in a pot-belly. Moreover, the amount of blood fat suddenly increases in the evening and, when asleep, one's blood flows more slowly and a large amount of blood fat is more easily deposited on the walls of blood vessels, increasing the danger of arteriosclerosis. This causes hypertension and coronary heart disease. Some patients of coronary heart disease die suddenly of myocardial infarction in sleep because they overeat greasy food at supper. Some died of acute necrotic pancreatitis for the same reason. So a folk saying goes, "Good breakfast, full lunch and light supper lead to long life."

Ran Dagu of Guangxi, 109 years old, said, "Take a good breakfast, a full lunch and a light supper. To work during the day you should eat plenty so you will be energetic. Since you rest in the evening, overeating at supper makes you feel like you are bulging." Rural inhabitants in eastern and northern Sichuan eat two meals a day. Even in families that take three meals a day, the elderly and children do not eat supper and other members eat a very simple supper. In summer they eat porridge and pickles and, in winter, noodles. Except for those doing heavy manual work, they generally eat only one bowl of porridge or noodles. On this diet, fat children and heavy old people are seldom seen in these areas. And, of course, they seldom suffer from cardiovascular diseases.

Family Harmony; Dutiful Posterity

Most Chinese centenarians live in families of warmth and harmony with the family as the centre of activities. These are families of four or five generations living together under one roof. With loving children and grandchildren, the old folks have spiritual sustenance and their lives are not lonesome. Therefore, the more they live, the longer they like to live on.

China has had the fine tradition of respecting the elderly since ancient times. Children and grandchildren take it as their obligation and duty to help old people live happily in their late years. Old people love and are solicitous about their children and grandchildren and try their best to share the worries of the family. Consequently, a warm, harmonious family takes shape.

The Chinese have great faith in the family concept and the family structure. This creats favourable conditions for the elderly to live peacefully in their late years and enjoy the happiness of a harmonious family, as most of Chinese centenarians are open-hearted and optimistic.

Grandma Song nee Shi, 103 years old, lives with her 77-year-old daughter in Dengyuan Township, Rugao County, Jiangsu Province. Sixteen family members of four generations have always lived together in harmony.

Grandma has never quarrelled with anyone. She is kind-hearted and all smiles to others. So local people call her "living Buddha with a smiling face." Although her family is not prosperous, her grandsons and granddaughters are very filial to her and ask her to eat first whatever delicious food they have. So Grandma leads a very happy life in her late years.

The tradition of family harmony and filial piety dominates in the cities as well as in the countryside. Zhu Shengwen, a retired engineer in Tianjin, has a happy family of four generations with one centenarian, all healthy in body and mind. Zhu Shengwen is 72 years old and his wife 65. He has a centenarian mother and five sons, three daughters, five daughters-in-law and seven grandsons. Respecting the old and loving the young, the family live in perfect harmony. The centenarian grandma remains good of hearing and vision and is sober and tranquil. Both Zhu and his wife, not yet white-haired, are in good health and walk with vigorous strides. The family was chosen as one of the municipal exemplary families in 1982 for family harmony and good relationship with neighbours.

Family harmony includes harmony between husband and wife. There are quite a number of married couples in China with both the husband and wife living to 100 years.

There is a married centenarian couple on Hongze Lake in Jiangsu Province. Grandpa Xue Tingzuo is 107 years old and his wife Xue nee Liu is 105. They moved from place to place in desperate circumstances in the old days and lost their only son. Though they lead a simple, plain life, they respect and take good care of each other. In this way they have lived together for more than 80 years. They are reverently called "old ancestors" by the villagers, who often bring them rice and firewood and carry water and sweep ground for them. In 1980 a feast was prepared in the village in celebration of Xue's 100th birthday and the 80th anniversary of the old couple's marriage.

There is a centenarian couple in Haodian Township, Yingshan County, Hubei Province. Grandpa Zeng Zhaohe is 104 years old and his wife Yu Shangying 106. Both Grandpa and Grandma, though white-haired, have ruddy and youthful complexion. They are healthy and can still do housework for themselves.

Yu Shangying came at the age of eight to Zeng Zhaohe's family as a child bride. They have lived happily together for nearly a century from childhood to a white-haired centenarian couple. Zeng Zhaohe is gentle and considerate. Yu Shangying is simple, diligent and devoted to her husband. Now the old couple live together happily and are inseparable as body and shadow. They are looking forward to the 100th anniversary of their wedding.

The longevity of this couple should also be attributed to the harmonious atmosphere of their family. Their son and daughter-in-law are both in their sixties and very filial to the old couple. They attend to the couple's needs in food, clothing, shelter and transportation with careful attention. In winter their daughter-in-law especially sews a suit of substantial but soft cotton-padded jacket and trousers for each of them. Their son and grandson gather firewood and make charcoal to make the old couple's room warm and snug. In summer their eldest granddaughter gives them sponge baths and helps move them to enjoy the cool under the tree shade. Their great granddaughter fans them and chases off mosquitoes. Seeing the children so filial, the old couple are always cheerful.

Local inhabitants and the government shower attentions on the old couple. Their neighbours often drop in for a visit. At festivals the juniors in the village call on them and bring the favourite foods of the old couple. The township government gives them a monthly subsidy and physicians of the township clinic give them regular physical check-ups. Thanks to the consideration of their family and the society, this centenarian couple live joyfully in the late years.

Longevity Linked to Heredity; Marry Late, Bear Few Children

Longevity, in general, is related to heredity. According to a survey in Hubei Province, 57 out of 88 centenarians have a history of long lives among family members. Heredity manifests itself more prominently among rural centenarians.

Grandpa Turdi Salay, 136 years old, of Yengisar County, Xinjiang, is China's oldest person. His family has three generations of centenarians. His mother died at the age of 110, his elder brother at the age of 135, one of his younger brothers at the age of 103 and another at the age of 101. His eldest daughter is now 110 years old and his youngest son is already 60.

This is a family of poor herdsmen. Turdi Salay had been a herdsman until he was 76. He was later hired by a merchant caravan and went with them to trade in Saudi Arabia, passing through Pakistan, India, Kashmir and Afghanistan along the ancient Silk Road. When he returned to his native land in 1948, he was already 100 years old.

Now his blood pressure and pulse are still normal and he can still climb upstairs. Only his left ear is slightly deaf. He and several of his family members constitute a family of centenarians, obviously attributable partly to heredity, but also because of good habits of regular manual work and sports participation, preference for sour milk and abstinence from smoking and drinking alcohol.

Centenarian Grandma Liu nee Zhang of Zhouba Township in Muchuan County, Sichuan Province, also has three generations of oldsters in her family. Her mother died at the age of 102 and her eldest sister lived to 103 years. Her daughter is almost 80 years old.

Centenarian Ma Gaze of Hui nationality on Qinghai Plateau lives in a family of five generations. Her mother died after reaching 100, and her eldest son and eldest daughter are both in their seventies.

But heredity is not the absolute factor in longevity. Born of the same parents of longevity, brothers and sisters do not necessarily all live long lives. Moreover, there are also cases in which parents attain longevity but their children are short-lived. Longevity is more closely related to one's care in preserving life—proper nutrition and proper balances between work and rest.

Hardships compelled quite a number of rural centenarians to marry late and bear few children, a circumstance that appears to have brought them good health and longevity.

Of 330 rural centenarians in Sichuan Province, ten men and four women married late, that is, after the age of 30. Six male centenarians married first between 40 and 50 and four others married first between 60 and 70, while four female centenarians had their first marriages after reaching 30. Eight male centenarians and three female centenarians remain single, most of them monks and nuns. Thirty-two female centenarians have never given birth and 23 bore only one child.

Eight rural centenarians in Sichuan married late, bore few or no children, or remain single, accounting for 24 percent of the total. Evidently, marrying late and bearing few children are not unfavourable to good health and longevity.

Bama Yao Autonomous County of Guangxi is the area of China most famous for the longevity of its people. Of the county's 150,000 inhabitants, 206 are in their nineties and 28 are centenarians. There are 18.7 centenarians per 100,000 people, the highest in China and close to the world's highest.

A survey of 18 centenarians showed five married first as teen-agers and another five marriages in their twenties. Eight had married first after reaching 30, including one who did not marry until 63.

Traditional Chinese medical theory holds that the essence of life stored in the kidneys plays a decisive role in determining life span. When one marries late, one better preserves the essence of life in the kidneys and therefore lives long, while others who are deficient in the essence of life in the kidneys live shorter lives. Whoever starts sexual activity too young will consume much of the essence of life in the kidneys. Those who marry late generally are temperate in their sex lives and will consume less of the essence of life in the kidneys, one explanation for longevity in those who marry late.

Marrying late and bearing few children implies that one should avoid over-indulgence in sex. Excessive sexual activity and too frequent emissions inevitably overburden men's testicles. Such activity also inhibits the secretion of the anterior of the pituitary gland, leading to atrophy of the testicles which, in turn, accelerates the onset of senility. Experiments show that animals with their testicles removed age very rapidly.

Too frequent emissions also cause massive loss of prostaglandin, which regulates the activities of the cardiovascular, respiratory and nervous systems and the function of the stomach and intestines. Prostaglandin deficiency will cause pathological changes and accelerate the senility of these organs. Semen also contains 0.2 percent of zinc, a trace element indispensable for the production of multiple proteins in the human body. Over-indulgence in sex hurts the kidneys and, in turn, shortens the life span.

Testicles of male oldsters begin to atrophy and deteriorate and the secretion of sex hormones begins to decline between ages 55 and 60. Other organs, such as heart, brain and kidney, also begin to grow old. Men who continue to indulge in sexual activity will inevitably accelerate their own senility, shortening their life spans. Therefore, marrying late and bearing few children, and especially temperance in sex, will help preserve the essence of life stored in the kidneys and prolong life.

Medicines to Strengthen Fragile Physique

Because most rural centenarians spent their early

lives in poverty, some are weak physically, and others have chronic ailments in varying degrees. They have prolonged their lives mainly by taking tonics, nourishing medicinal herbs. Centenarian Grandma Dang nee Jiang of Wenfeng Township in Nanchong County, Sichuan Province used to be a very fat woman. She got seriously ill at the age of 60 and became emaciated. A local veteran told her a secret prescription: one or two crucian carp each day, steamed with 10 grams each of sweet almonds and the seed powder of Gorgon fruit. After eating crucian carp for three months she gradually developed in physical strength. She has eaten this preparation 20 to 30 times each year to achieve good health. Her white hair has turned black, her complexion is ruddy and she is still able to do light chores.

Almonds were the main ingredient for preventing aging in ancient prescriptions. Current studies show the almond contains vitamin B17, which can promote the regeneration of cells. The seeds of Gorgon fruit are excellent for strengthening the spleen and nourishing the kidneys and can also improve the function of the immune system. These two complement to the high-protein crucian carp. Together they strengthen the spleen, nourish the kidneys, build the physique and delay senility.

Guangxi, Guizhou and Sichuan abound in medicinal herbs which rural inhabitants use to build their physiques, nourish deficiencies and prevent and treat diseases. Most medicinal herbs are neither toxic nor have unfavourable side effects. Since they have the convenience of being collected locally, a considerable number of centenarians have never taken pharmaceuticals in their lives. When they suffer from minor injuries or

93

ailments, they often gather medicinal herbs to treat themselves.

Bama Yao Autonomous County in Guangxi, a home of longevity, abounds in sealwort (*Polygonatum sibiricum*) and clams. Having eaten sealwort and clams over a long time, many centenarians are healthy and strong and seldom suffer from severe diseases. Thanks to sealwort and clam, which are both tonic and nourishing, quite a number of old people are still capable of sexual activity at 80 and some even intend to marry at the age of 90.

Centenarian Grandma Chen nee Tian of Guizhou Province gathers wild medicinal herbs both to treat her own ailments and to serve fellow villagers. She has become a sparetime rural physician, skilled in the use of wild medicinal herbs.

Sichuan Province ranks first in China for its aboundance of medicinal herbs. Many rural centenarians can identify a dozen wild medicinal herbs and know quite a number of folk prescriptions. Some folk prescriptions, costing next to nothing, can cure diseases that have been treated without success by major hospitals.

Zeng Yulian (101) of Leshan, Li Shuqing (102) and Luo Huiming (100) of Emei County, Lü Fuqian (100) of Meishan County and Yu Haiqing (102) of Guangyuan County, all of Sichuan Province, treat diseases in others with wild medicinal herbs.

Some people often eat tonic, nourishing medicinal herbs to achieve longevity. Grandpa Yuan Kaixing, 106 years old, lives in Pinggang Village in Yuanshan Township, Pingchang County, Sichuan Province. At 24 he left his native village for Taibai Mountains in Shaanxi Province to gather medicinal herbs. He drank spring water and ate the root of straight ladybell (*Adenophora stricta*), Chinese yam and sealwort. He seldom had chance to eat rice and wheat flour. He did not return to his native Yuanshan Township until he was 65, and had long been in the habit of eating medicinal herbs as substitutes for cereals. After returning home, he has often eaten Chinese yam and the root of straight ladybell as his meal. Now he is 106 years old but still has good hearing and vision and speaks clearly. Walking or climbing hills, he races young people and can carry buckets with 25 kilograms of water for 30 kilometres.

A rural centenarian in Hunan Province likes to eat a kind of wild fruit. He is in the habit of eating this fruit when he works in the mountains every day. He has never taken other medicines and attributes his good health and longevity to eating this fruit. The Hunan Provincial Institute of Traditional Chinese Medicine and Pharmacology is now studying the anti-senility elements of this fruit.

The above-mentioned incidents demonstrate that some natural plants indeed contain medicines for prolonging life. These plants may be very ordinary and easy to get, not as rare and expensive as ginseng root.

It has also been noticed that those with fragile physiques or who are afflicted with chronic minor ailments and often take medicines may live long, while death may find an easy prey in those who seem to be healthy and strong and free of any disease. This signifies to the effect of medicines. Those weak in constitution pay constant attention to the art of healthy living, taking medicines whenever necessary. Consequently, they are in a position to survive severe diseases and therefore live long. On the other hand, one who is strong in physique and not susceptible to minor ailments may not take proper care of himself in daily life. When he suddenly falls ill, his life is endangered.

Service to Others; Virtue

Most Chinese centenarians are honest, kind-hearted and willing to help and render service to others.

Although most rural centenarians were born of poor families, they take their poverty with good grace and remain contented and peaceful in mind. They are charitable and often help one another over financial difficulties. When disaster falls upon one family, all others offer help. They seem willing to give whatever they possess to help those in need, although their own families are very poor.

Centenarian physician Luo Mingshan of Sichuan Province used to practise medicine among ordinary people. As he had a secret prescription "one-hundred-herb pill" handed down through generations in his family to go with his excellent medical skills, many patients came to him for treatment. He treated free of charge those who were too poor to pay and helped with their food and lodging. He was generous with poor peasants who were in financial straits.

One year his pharmacy was swept away by a mountain flood taking all his possessions. In the midst of this misfortune a patient called on Luo and complained that his house had caught fire and was burnt to ashes and he could no longer earn his livelihood, not to mention afford medical treatment. Luo instantly gave this stranger patient his three remaining silver dollars.

In the depth of one winter Luo saw a patient wearing only two unlined jackets, so he took off his own cotton-padded waistcoat to give the patient. Luo often pays lodging expenses for patients who have come from a distance. Generous towards others, he himself is very frugal in daily life, eating simple meals and wearing homemade clothes. He is therefore known in his hometown as "Kindness Luo."

There are many examples of centenarian physicians like Luo Mingshan. In Jixin Township of Fenghuang County in Hunan Province there is a 106-year-old physician named Tian Zhongshun, who has practised medicine gratis for 90 years, beginning at the age of 16. Even after he was employed by the state, medicinal herbs from his home herbal garden have been offered to patients free of charge. Patients who call on him in his off hours, on holidays or at festivals are treated without charge. Since his retirement at the age of 96, Tian has continued to grow medicinal herbs or to go into the hills to gather herbs and has treated patients without charge. He has stipulated three rules for himself: First, do not practise favouritism for relatives or friends. Second, do not accept gifts from patients. Third, treat all patients alike and do not give preferential treatment to patients of higher status or greater wealth.

Tian has practised medicine for nine decades and taught 30 disciples. Under his guidance, his children and grandchildren also practise medicine free of charge. He once said, "When I see my effort can alleviate patient sufferings, I enjoy a kind of indescribable happiness. I feel very content."

Physician Chen Zhao, 101 years old, of Xingren Township in Nantong County, Jiangsu Province and

Tang Daocheng, a retired veteran herbal preparer of Biyang County in Henan Province have both treated fellow villagers and townsmen free of charge. Because of their selfless effort to help others, they are well-known and highly respected among the local people.

Willingness to help others is fairly common among Chinese centenarians. Grandma Ye Genlian, 109 years old, lives in a village on Chengdu's outskirts. Skilled at making cloth shoes, she often does needlework for others. Many believe that one who wears a pair of shoes made by persons of longevity will himself live a long life. Therefore many villagers have asked her to make shoes for them, which she does, declaring that "seeing others wear the shoes I make, I feel joy."

Liu Qinghe, 100 years old, of Dayi County, western Sichuan, was born to a peasant family in Pengxi County 500 kilometres away in the northern part of the province. Before Liberation he was a hired hand. He is always ready to take up the cudgels for a just cause, helping the weak against the powerful. He always does his best to help anyone whose family has fallen into trouble. He said, "One must be good both inside and outside. First of all, he should be good-hearted. If he is vicious in heart, conditions of his body will change for the worse; but if he is good in heart and morals, his body and internal organs will all be in good condition." This complies with the ancient saying that "the virtuous attain longevity," and it applies to both rural and urban centenarians.

Professor Ma Yinchu fought for truth all his life. In the 1940s he worked with all his might againt Japanese aggression. In the 1950s he spoke out for population control, which ran against Mao Zedong's slogans. In the

60s, when knowledge was regarded as useless by many people in China because of political turmoil, Ma tried his best to popularize science. He remained unyielded when he suffered persecution in the 70s, and in the 80s he reached his 100th birthday.

Centenarian calligrapher Sun Mofo also paid great attention to moral cultivation. He took "do deeds of merit, be virtuous, expound ideas in writing and achieve great benevolence, wisdom and courage" as his motto, often writing it for young friends to encourage them. As a brave, intelligent young man he had followed Sun Yat-sen in bringing bourgeois revolution. In old age he worked hard for the benefit of society. He spent decades writing 500 copies of *The Art of Chinese Calligraphy* (*Shu Pu*, a book on how to practise calligraphy by Sun Guoting of the Tang Dynasty) and gave them to various libraries and colleges in China. He also presented 3,000 vertical scrolls of his calligraphy to cultural and educational institutions. He was always ready to write calligraphical scrolls for anyone who asked for them, never taking any rewards or gifts in return. He said, "One should first of all be virtuous. Persons of virtue attain longevity. A person of high moral principles remains tranquil in mind and sound in body. It is only natural that he lives long."

Traditional Chinese Body-Building Art

Body-building exercises have a long history in China. Their emphasis on mental cultivation or the training of consciousness has made them unique in world culture. The regulation of breathing is the most important means to achieve mental concentration.

Mawangdui *Daoyin* Exercises

This set of *daoyin* exercises was worked out by Tong Junjie of Hunan Provincial College of Traditional Chinese Medicine from a coloured silk painting unearthed from a 2,000-year-old Western Han tomb at Mawangdui Village on Changsha's outskirts in Hunan Province (Fig.). The painting depicts over 40 men and women variously dressed and in different postures, mostly barehanded, but some with weapons. Methods inscribed on a bronze mirror excavated from a Western Han tomb were also incorporated into this set of exercises, which has proved effective through years of practice. It has now become widely popularized in China.

Mawangdui *daoyin* exercises consist of six steps.

Step one. Stand quietly in a calm state of mind with clothes and belt loosened, the tip of the tongue touching the upper palate behind the teeth. Overlap hands on

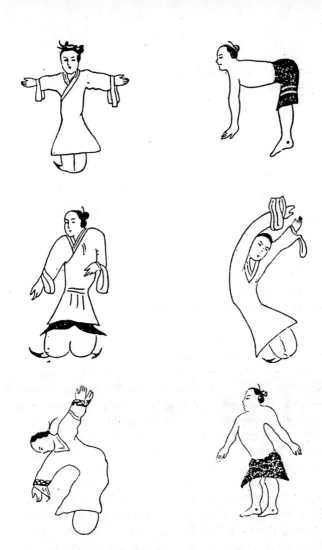

Daoyin **Exercises on a Silk Painting Unearthed at Mawangdui**

stomach, or the area below the navel, known as *dantian*. Men put left hand over right hand, women put right hand over the left. Relax the entire body, draw the chin in slightly, place feet parallel and shoulder-width apart (Fig. 1). Close the eyes to allow only a slit of light to pass. Concentrate thought at point *zuqiao* between the eyes, gaze afar and roll eyes eight times. Then regulate breathing, contract the anus when inhaling and (in imagination) direct *qi* to point *mingmen* at the second lumbar vertebra, just opposite the navel. When exhaling, direct *qi*

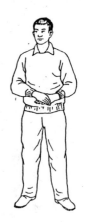

Figure 1

from *dantian* to point *huiyin* (in the centre of the perineum between the anus and the sex organs). Repeat this exercise nine times. Then count breath from one to nine silently three times, clearing the mind of all thoughts. Listen to the sound of breathing for three minutes. Next, imagine that *dantian* is pressed against *mingmen*, *mingmen* is pressed against *baihui* (in the middle on top of the head) and *baihui* is pressed against *dantian*. Repeat this thought sequence three times. Then go to step two.

Step two. Circulate *qi* inside the body. Touch the upper palate behind teeth with tongue. Direct *qi* to point *huiyin* while contracting the anus-lifting muscle. When *qi* can be felt at *huiyin*, direct it to *weilü* (coccyx), *mingmen*, *jizhong* (at the 11th lumbar vertebra), *dazhui* (at the seventh cervical vertebra, the high bone on the nape), *yuzhen* (central point on occipital bone) and

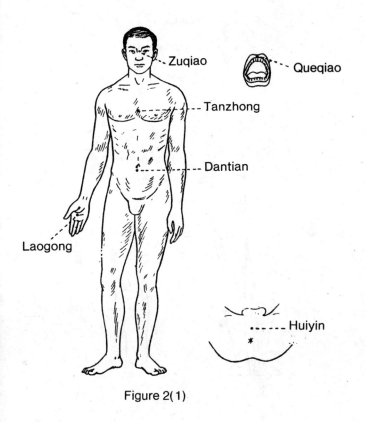

Figure 2(1)

baihui. Rotate the *qi* around *baihui*, clockwise for male and counter-clockwise for female. Then move it from *baihui* across *zuqiao*, the tongue, *tanzhong* (midway between the two nipples), *dantian*, *huiyin* and *yongquan* (on the balls of the feet) (Fig.2). Repeat this three times. After it circles around *baihui* for the third time, pass the

103

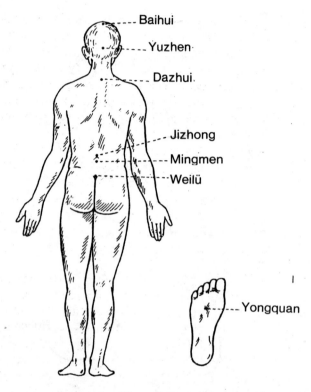

Figure 2(2)

qi to *dantian* and concentrate the mind on *dantian*. Take no heed of sounds, sights and smells in the surroundings.

Step three. Shake the head slightly to loosen the neck. Move the hands from *dantian* to a spread position as if holding a large balloon, left hand moving downward and right hand upward (Fig. 3), and meanwhile rotate body to the right slowly. Then turn left, with left hand moving upward and right hand downward. Repeat the movement nine times. Then move the arms slowly out to the side, in gentle waving motions, with the elbows slightly bent, for a moment before returning hands to *dantian*, folding the arms in as a red-crown crane takes in its wings.

Step four. Stand in the same posture as in step one, but with both palms turned upward and fingertips touching at *dantian* (Fig. 4). On hot days think of snowflakes whirling in the sky and on cold days envision a gush of hot spring water from *baihui* on top of the head cascading down the face, upper limbs and chest. Slip into a state of relaxation, happiness and contentment.

Step five. Let the tongue touch upper palate behind the teeth; thrust the head forward and draw it back; tap teeth together, and press middle finger (Fig. 5) against *dantian* 36 times. (Males use left middle finger; females use right middle finger.) Then lick the upper palate and the inside and outside of the teeth to stimulate saliva secretion. Divide the saliva in the mouth into three small gulps and swallow them, guiding (in imagination) the first portion to the throat, the second to *tanzhong* and the third to *dantian*.

Step six. Stand in a natural posture with weight on the heels, with closed eyes and hands at the sides (Fig. 6). Imagine oneself in the woods of a quiet hill; let the body sway as gently as willow branches rustling in a breeze. Meanwhile, think of this verse,

In the stillness of night all worries are gone,

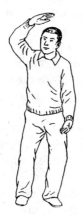

Figure 3

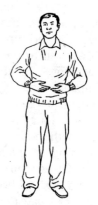

Figure 4

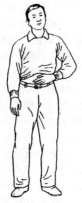

Figure 5

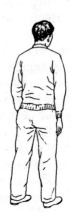

Figure 6

My whole body relaxes and sways with the wind.
My thoughts hold closely to dantian with seven aper-
tures in the head sealed,
I feel happy and content, soaring lightly into the sky.

At this time if the body wants to move, let it move to its natural inclination. If it does not want to move, do not press for motion, just allow things to take their own course; be relaxed and at ease. Stay in this state for half an hour before beginning the conclusion of the exercise.

How to conclude: Concentrate the thought on point *yongquan* on the balls of the feet. Think repeatedly: "I am going to conclude the exercise. I am going to stop." Should one fail to stop, press the middle of the ring finger with thumb or press point *jianjing* (the highest point on the shoulder-collarbone joint). If necessary, open the eyes for a moment and the body's movement will gradually stop. When the body is still, bring the hands from the sides and place them close together at *dantian* before raising them gently above the chest to the chin (Fig. 7). Then rotate the hands to palms-up beside the cheekbones (Fig. 8) and concentrate thought on the tips of the middle fingers. Then direct *qi* and blood with one's thought while massaging the point *baihui* nine times. Men massage with left hand clockwise and women massage with right hand counter-clockwise. Then massage palms and backs of hands until they are warm, massage the face and head in a combining motion with the fingers 36 times in a sequence of face, top and back of head. Walk slowly between 30 and 50 paces and concentrate *qi* into *dantian*. Now, the full set of *daoyin* exercises has been concluded.

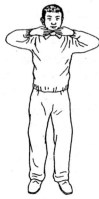

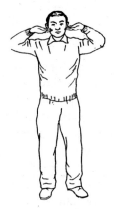

Figure 7   Figure 8

Five-Animal Games

The Five-Animal Games are a set of *daoyin* exercise worked out by Hua Tuo, a famous physician of the Eastern Han Dynasty, imitating the movements of tiger, deer, bear, ape and bird. Hua Tuo often practised these games, and "looked young and robust when he was nearly a hundred years old." His disciple Wu Pu, who also practised the Five-Animal Games as a daily habit, lived into his 90s and remained "good of hearing and vision and with a complete set of firm teeth." This illustrates the benefits of the games to health and longevity.

The Five-Animal Games were gradually developed and improved over a thousand years. In the Ming Dynasty they were reconstituted as standing postures replaced seated ones. Its different sections were linked into a complete set and techniques from Indian callisthenics were included. A brief account of the games follows, accompanied by diagrams recorded in *Chi Feng Sui*, a book on *qigong* by Zhou Lüjing of the Ming Dynasty.

The tiger game (Fig.1): Hold breath, bow the head slightly and rotate the fists, standing in a hunched posture as of a tiger in a fury. The two hands feel as if they are easily lifting a thousand *jin* (five hundred kilograms) of iron. Still holding the breath, straighten

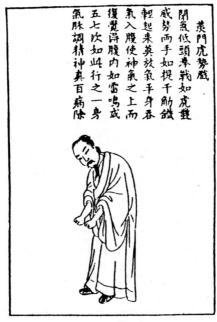

The Tiger Game

the body and propel the breath deep into the abdomen, making it rise and descend as a thunderous roar develops in the abdomen. Repeat this seven times. This can bring harmony of *qi* and blood to refresh the mind and eliminate diseases.

The bear game (Fig. 2): Hold breath, clench fists, and stand sideways like a bear with the right fist lifted upward and the left fist held low to the left. Move the feet left and right, forward and backward in a type of

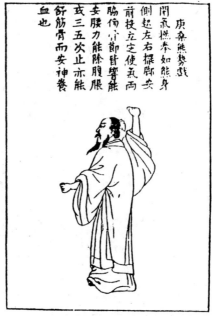

The Bear Game

slow dance step. Direct *qi* from the armpits across the joints until all joints tingle with the effort. Repeat three to five times. This can increase lower back strength, reduce abdominal distension, relax tendons and bones, calm the mind and nourish the blood.

The deer game (Fig.3): Hold breath, lower head, clench fists and turn the head slightly as a deer would to look at its tail. Straighten the body with shoulders squared, rising on the tips of the toes. Vibrate throughout the body from the heels to the neck. Repeat three

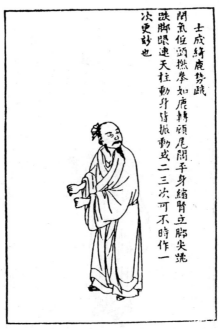

The Deer Game

times. It is best to do this game from time to time.

The ape game (Fig.4): Hold breath and simulate climbing up a tree like an ape, as one hand rotates in a movement of twirling a fruit, with one raised foot, turn on the heel of the other, directing the *qi* and swallowing it into the abdomen. Repeat the movement left and right alternately until the body begins to sweat.

The bird game (Fig.5): Hold breath and make the movement of a bird ready to take its flight, extending the arms outward to the sides and gently moving them over the head. Direct *qi* from *weilü* (coccyx) up the

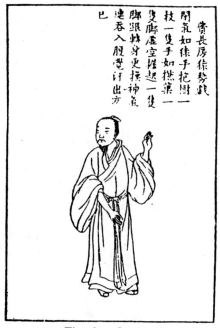

The Ape Game

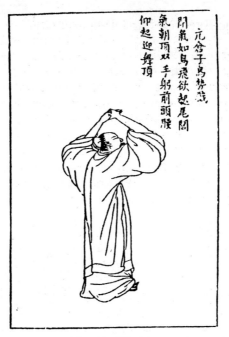

元像子鳥勢戲

閉氣如鳥飛欲起尾閭
氣朝頂以手躬前頭腰
仰起迎舞頂

The Bird Game

spine to the top of the head. Raise hands to clasp a few inches above the head, raise head and lower back as hands move up and down as though flying.

Each individual should adapt these exercises to his own conditions. It is important not only to mimic the external movements of the five animals but also to reflect their habits and expressions. Relax and be at ease, effortless and effective. Pay attention to the cultivation of the *qi* and spirit.

Brocade Exercises in Twelve Forms

The brocade exercises in eight forms first appeared in *Essentials of Preserving Life* (*She Sheng Yao Yi*) written in the Song Dynasty. They became widespread in Ming times. In the Qing Dynasty Pan Wei, a scholar on the art of healthy living, using medical literiture for reference, revised the routines, turning them into the brocade exercises in twelve forms.

In 1854 Wang Zuyuan, another scholar on the art of healthy living, stayed for over three months in Shaolin Monastery, where he saw a diagram of exercises similar to Pan Wei's twelve forms. Wang did the exercises on the diagram for over four decades with excellent results. He published the diagram with explanations.

Step one. Sit with legs crossed and eyes firmly closed. Clear the mind of distracting thoughts. When sitting, spinal column should be straight; lower back should be relaxed and the body must not lean against anything. Firmly clench both hands. Meditate in this way to preserve tranquility of the mind.

Step two. Tap teeth together lightly 36 times, making a distinct clicking sound each time. This serves to concentrate the mind so it will not be distracted. Interlock the fingers of both hands behind the head and pull them snugly to the nape of the neck, holding the ears flat with the palms. Silently count nine breaths through the nose, breathing lightly without sound.

Step three. After counting nine breaths inhaled and exhaled, separate hands and move palms further apart to cover both ears. Place forefingers on middle fingers and then vigorously tap the back of the head with forefingers, sounding to the ears like beats on a drum,

闭目冥心坐，握固静思神，

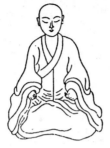

第 一 图

盘腿而坐，紧闭两目，冥亡心中杂念。凡坐要竖起脊梁，腰不可软弱，身不可倚靠。握固者，握手牢固，可以闭关切邪也；静思者，静息思虑而存神也。

Figure 1

叩齿三十六，两手抱昆仑，

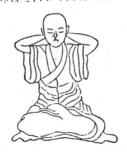

第 二 图

上下牙齿，相叩作响，宜三十六声，叩齿以集身内之神使不散也。昆仑即头，以两手十指相叉，抱住后颈，即用两手掌紧掩耳门，暗记鼻息九次，微微呼吸，不宜有声。

Figure 2

24 times on each side. Then put both hands in the lap, grasping them firmly together.

Step four. Lower the head, turn it to look sidewise, first to the left and then to the right, bringing shoulders forward accordingly, right shoulder for left look, left for right. Repeat 24 times each side.

Step five. Let the tongue touch the upper palate before moving it around the inside of the mouth 36 times to produce saliva; rinse the mouth with it. Swallow the saliva in three gulps with gurgling sounds. Imagine the saliva, accompanied by *qi*, flows from the throat to *dantian*.

Step six. Take a deep breath and hold it. Rub palms together until they are very warm, then press hands against spots on both sides of the lower spinal column, massaging while exhaling slowly. Massage the two soft spots beside the lower back 26 times. Put hands down to sides and firmly clench fists.

Step seven. Hold breath and concentrate the mind in meditation. Imagine a flame in the heart spreading downward to the region of *dantian* until the whole body feels warm. Then exhale through the nose.

Step eight. Bring both hands to the square in front of the body. Put left hand on right shoulder and pull, twisting the trunk to the left 36 times as if turning a windlass. Repeat with the right hand on the left shoulder.

Step nine. Stretch the legs straight out in front of the body. Lock hands together with fingers, palms up. First put the interlocked hands above the head, then push them up as if lifting a heavy stone, making a special effort to stiffen and raise and straighten the lower back. Relax by bringing hands onto the head and repeat the

左右鸣天鼓，二十四度闻，

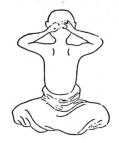

第 三 图

记算鼻息出入各九次毕。即放所叉之手。移两手掌擦耳。以第二指叠在中指上。作力放下第二指。重弹脑后。要如击鼓之声。左右各二十四度。两手同弹。共四十八声。仍放手握固。

Figure 3

微摆撼天柱，

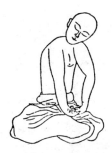

第 四 图

天柱即后颈，低头扭颈向左右侧视，肩亦随之左右招摆，各二十四次。

Figure 4

赤龙搅水津，鼓漱三十六，神水满口匀，
一口分三咽，龙行虎自奔；

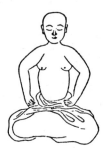

第 五 图

赤龙即舌，以舌顶上腭，又搅满口内上下两旁，使水津
自生，鼓漱于口中三十六次。神水即津液，分作三次，要汩
汩有声吞下。心暗想，口嗓舌，所存津液，直送至脐下丹田。
龙即津，虎即气，津下去，气自随之。

Figure 5

闭气搓手热，背摩后精门，

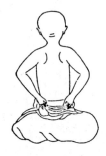

第 六 图

以鼻吸气闭之，用两掌相搓擦极热，急分两手磨后腰上
两边，一面徐徐放气从鼻出。精门即后腰两边软处，以两手
磨二十六遍，仍收手握固。

Figure 6

118

尽此一口气，想火烧脐轮，

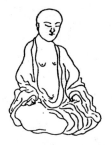

第 七 图

闭口鼻之气，以心暗想，运心头之火，下烧丹田，觉似有热，仍放气从鼻出。脐轮即脐丹田。

Figure 7

左右辘轳转，

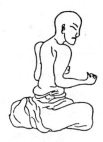

第 八 图

曲湾两手。先以左手连肩。凹转三十六次。如绞车一般。右手亦如之。此单转辘轳法。

Figure 8

两脚放舒伸，叉手双虚托，

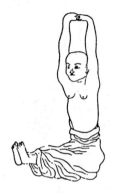

第 九 图

放所盘两脚，平伸向前，两手指相叉，反掌向上，先安所叉之手于头顶，作力上托，要如重石在手，托上腰身，俱著力上耸。手托上一次，又放下安手头顶，又托上。共九次。

Figure 9

低头攀足频，

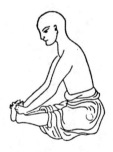

第 十 图

以两手向所伸两脚底作力扳之，头低如礼拜状。十二次，仍收足盘坐，收手握固。

Figure 10

以候神水至，再漱再吞津，如此三度毕，
神水九次吞，咽下汩汩响，百脉自调匀，

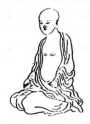

第 十 一 图
再用舌搅口内，以候神水满口，再鼓漱三十六。连前一
度，此再两度，共三度毕，前一度作三次吞，此两度作六次
吞，共九次，吞如前。咽下要汩汩响声，咽津三度，百脉自
周遍调匀。

Figure 11

河车搬运毕，想发火烧身；旧名八段锦，
子后午前行，勤行无间断，万疾化为尘。

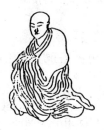

第 十 二 图
心想脐下丹田中，似有热气如火，闭气如忍大便状，将
热气运至谷道，即大便处，升上腰间，背脊后颈，脑后头顶
止。又闭气，从额上两太阳，耳根前，两面颊，降至喉下，
心窝肚脐下丹田止。想是发火烧，通身皆热。

Figure 12

121

process. Do it nine times.

Step ten. Stretch the hands forward to grasp firmly the balls of the extended feet and lower the head as if paying homage. Repeat 12 times. Return to a crossed leg position; place clenched fists on lap.

Step eleven. Again move the tongue in the mouth until the saliva accumulates and rinse the mouth by swishing the saliva around 36 times. This has been done once before (step five) and now do it twice. In all, do it three times, swallowing a total of nine gulps.

Step twelve. Concentrate the mind on *dantian*, where warm *qi* burns. Hold breath as if trying to hold back a bowel movement and direct the warm *qi* at *dantian* to the anus. Then raise the *qi* to the lower back, spinal column, neck, back of the head and up to the top of the head. Again hold breath and let the *qi* descend from the temples to the front of the ears, cheeks, throat, chest and down to *dantian*. Imagine a fire that burns vigorously in *dantian*, sending warmth to all parts of the body.

Limbering Exercises for Tendons

The origin of the limbering exercises for tendons is uncertain, though they have long been attributed to Bodhidharma of Shaolin Monastery, founder of the Chan school of Buddhism in China. They have been handed down as one of the many boxing styles of the Shaolin Monastery. It is said that Yue Fei, a Song Dynasty military hero, used these exercises to train his formidable troops. Since then, they have become widespread among the people.

Step one. Wei Tuo presenting a club (1).

Stand erect and look straight ahead. Cup one hand in the other in front of the chest as if grasping a club in the hands. Show absorbed attention and a modest attitude as though presenting a club to an elder.

Step two. Wei Tuo presenting a club (2).

Stand on tiptoe, arms outstretched to the sides, palms down. Breathe slowly and evenly, look straight ahead and focus the attention on a point.

Step three. Wei Tuo presenting a club (3).

Stand on tiptoe, arms upraised, with palms up and eyes looking upward as if to see an object on the hands. Stand with legs stiffened. Clench the teeth, touch the upper palate with the tongue and breathe through nose. Let the brain rest, then clench fists, put them slowly to

韦驮献杵第一势　　　　　　韦驮献杵第二势

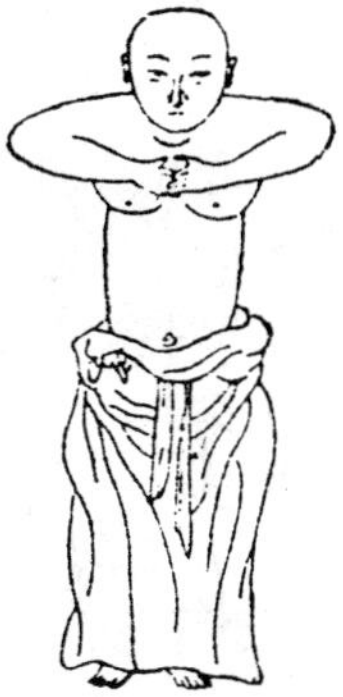

立身期正直，环拱手当胸，
气定神皆敛，心澄貌亦恭。

Figure 1

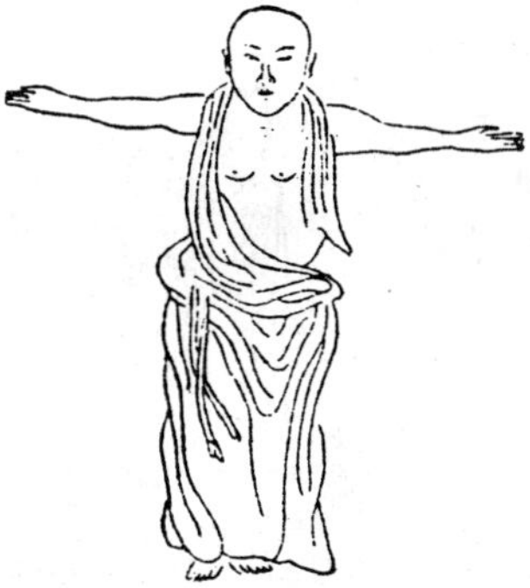

足指挂地，两手平开，
心平气静，目瞪口呆。

Figure 2

the sides and lower heels on the ground.

Step four. Lifting hands to pluck stars.

Put the left hand on lower back while lifting the right hand as if striving to pluck a star, with palm above the head and eyes looking at the raised hand. Inhale through the nose while drawing the raised hand vigorously back to the side. Then use the left hand to repeat the movement.

Step five. Pulling nine oxen by the tail.

Take a big step forward with left foot, bending the left leg at knee and straightening the right leg, with the

韦驮献杵第三势

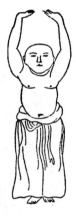

掌托天门目上观，足尖著地立身端，
力周骹胁浑如植，咬紧牙关不放宽，
舌可生津将腭抵，鼻能调息觉心安，
两拳缓缓收回处，用力还将挟重看。

Figure 3

摘星换斗势

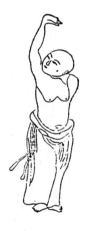

只手擎天掌覆头，更从掌内注双眸，
鼻端吸气频调息，用力收回左右侔。

Figure 4

body leaning slightly forward. Direct the *qi* of the lower abdomen up into arms. Put the left hand in front as if grasping the tail of an ox, give a vigorous pull, fixing both eyes on the left hand. Alternate left and right in doing this movement.

Step six. Extending claws and flapping wings.

Stand with chest raised. Stare ahead with angry eyes. Thrust hands forward at chest level and draw them back vigorously, repeating the movement seven times.

Step seven. Nine ghosts pulling a sabre.

Encircle the head with the right hand and pull to the right vigorously. Repeat with the left hand. Do this several times.

Step eight. Planting feet on the ground in a triangle.

Touch upper palate with the tongue, eyes wide open,

出爪亮翅势

倒拽九牛尾势

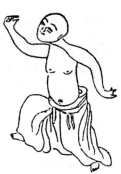

两腿后伸前屈，小腹运气空松，
用力在于两膀，观拳须往双瞻。

Figure 5

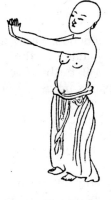

挺身兼怒目，推手向当前，
用力收回处，功须七次全。

Figure 6

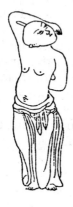

九鬼拔马刀势

側首弯肱，抱顶及頸，自头收回，
弗嫌力猛，左右相轮，身直气静。

Figure 7

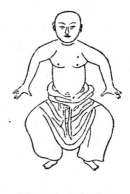

三盘落地势

上腭坚撑舌，张眸意注牙，
足开蹲似踞，手按猛如拏；
两掌翻齐起，千觔重有加，
瞪睛兼闭口，起立足无斜。

Figure 8

teeth clenched. Drop to a half squat until thighs are nearly parallel to the ground. Move the hands downward as if pushing something into the ground. Then turn palms up as if holding up a heavy object. Repeat three times.

Step nine. Blue dragon extending its claws.

Stand upright, eyes straight ahead, left hand clenched into fist beside the hipbone at the waist and with fingers of the fist up. Stretch right hand, palm down, across the chest to the left, pushing strength into the hand. Swinging the hand low to skirt the knee, return it to the side. Place the right fist at the waist and use the left hand for the movement across the chest. As the hands move, breathe evenly and be calm in mind. Repeat several times, alternating left and right.

Step ten. A tiger grabbing at prey.

Fall forward to place fingers of both hands on the ground, bend left leg forward at the knee and straighten right leg to extend behind the body. Hold head up and thrust the chest forward. With the body straining forward, breathe evenly. Then reverse the process, placing right foot forward and straightening the left leg. Repeat several times.

Step eleven. Bowing low.

Stand with feet apart. Hold the back of the head with interlocked fingers. Draw the abdomen in, bend at the waist, bend the head downward as far as it will go, preferably until it is between the thighs. Close the mouth, clench the teeth and let the tip of the tongue

青龙探爪势

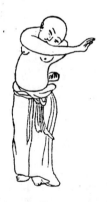

青龙探爪，左从右出，修士效之，掌平气实；
力周肩背，围收过膝，两目注平，息调心注。

Figure 9

卧虎扑食势

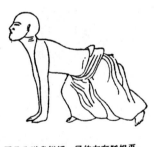

两足分跺身似倾，屈伸左右骸相更，
昂头胸作探前势，偃背腰还似骶平；
鼻息调元均出入，指尖著地赖支撑，
降龙伏虎神仙事，学得真形也卫生。

Figure 10

touch the upper palate. Breathe through the nose. Then straighten up to bend forward again. Repeat several times.

Step twelve. Twisting the tail.

Interlock hands and bend waist until palms are on the ground. Hold head up, open eyes widely and gaze straight ahead while stamping the feet. Stand up and repeat the process 21 times. Then spread the forearms to the sides seven times. Finally sit straight with crossed legs. Close eyes slightly and regulate the breathing to an even cadence. Concentrate the mind at *dantian* and enter into a quiescent mental state.

掉 尾 势

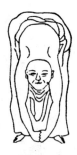

打 躬 势

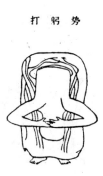

两手齐持脑，垂腰至膝间，
头惟探胯下，口更齿牙关，
掩耳聪教塞，调元气自闲，
舌尖还抵腭，力在肘双弯。

Figure 11

膝直膀伸，推手自地，瞪目昂头，
凝神壹志，起而顿足，二十一次，
左右伸肱，以七为志，更作坐功，
盘膝垂眦，口注于心，息调于鼻，
定静乃起，厥功维备，总考其法，
图成十二，谁实贻诸，五代之季，
达摩西来，传少林寺，有宋岳侯，
更为鉴识，却病延年，功无与类。

Figure 12

Daoyin Curative Arts of Ancients of Longevity

Each famous Chinese ancient of longevity had his own special *daoyin* method for healing diseases. These valuable experiences have always been prized. Survival of the *daoyin* arts to the present is a testimony to their practical value.

From among nearly 200 ancient diagrams, 16 are selected here. They prevent and heal common elderly ailments such as headache, blurred vision, chest and abdominal pains, heart ache, lumbago and leg pain, hemiplegia, seminal emission and general debility. Each

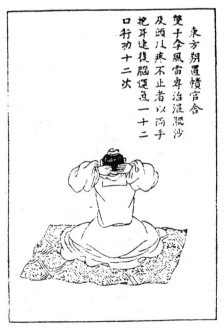

東方朔置幘宮舍
雙手今風帝身治混照沙
及兩肤疼不止者以兩手
把耳連提脇運氣一十二
口行功十二次

Figure 1

of these exercises is attributed to a famous immortal or scholar, gaining widespread acceptance.

Dongfang Shuo's method of healing severe headache (Fig. 1): Hold ears and back of the head with hands. Breathe evenly, exhaling through the mouth 12 times. Concentrate the mind at *dantian* and direct *qi* into *dantian* when inhaling through nose. Remove hands from head and start over. Repeat 12 times. This method heals acute attacks of chronic headache, including nervous, vascular and hypertensive headaches.

Rong Chenggong's method of healing dizziness (Fig. 2): Clench teeth and hold breath. Press ears with palms

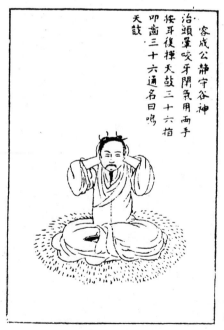

Figure 2

and tap at the back of the head with forefingers 36 times; then tap teeth lightly 36 times. This exercise is also called "beating the heavenly drum." It serves to heal various types of dizziness caused by hypertension, Meniere's syndrome and vehicle and boat sickness.

Kou Xian's method of healing pain and stiffness of the head and the neck (Fig. 3): Press knees separately with hands. Turn head, neck and back to the left. Exhale

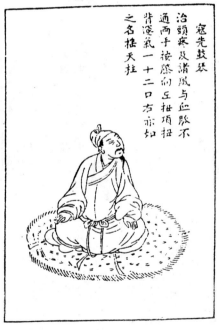

Figure 3

through mouth 12 times at the same time. Then turn head, neck and back right and also exhale through mouth 12 times. This exercise is called "shaking the heavenly pillar." It serves to heal pain and stiffness of head and neck, including nervous headache, disease of cervical vertebrae and headache caused by hypertension.

Zi Zhu's method of healing dizziness (Fig. 4): Sit upright. First rub soles with hands until they become warm. Then press knees with hands and exhale through mouth nine times. This heals blurred vision and feelings

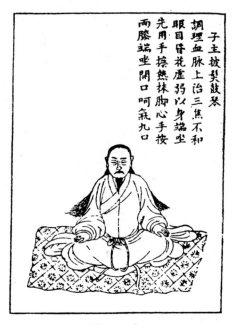

Figure 4

of top heaviness, various chronic diseases of the eyes and arteriosclerosis in the eye area caused by hypertension.

Xu Jingyang's method of healing heart pain (Fig. 5): Stand with right foot behind and pointing to the right. Raise right hand, turn torso and eyes to the left. Put left hand behind the lower body and exhale through the mouth nine times, inhaling into *dantian*. This heals all types of heart pain including angina pectoris of coron-

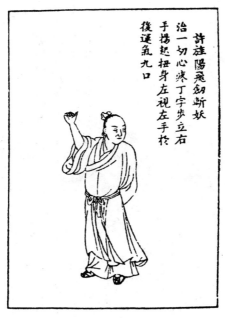

許旌陽飛釵斷妖
治一切心疼丁字步立右
手揚起扭身左視左手於
後運氣九口

Figure 5

ary heart disease and stomach trouble.

Tao Chenggong's method of healing congestion and discomfort in chest and diaphragm (Fig. 6): Elevate and extend both hands to the left while turning head to the right, then put the hands to the right and turn the head left, exhaling through mouth nine times in each position. This serves to heal congestion and discomfort at the chest, including tracheitis and emphysema.

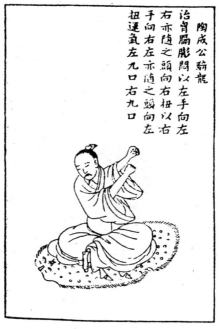

Figure 6

Fu Lü's method of healing abdominal pains (Fig. 7): Sit upright and close eyes slightly. Clasp *dantian* with hands. Exhale through mouth 49 times, inhaling through nose into *dantian*. This exercise serves to heal abdominal pains caused by chronic gastritis, ulcers and chronic colitis.

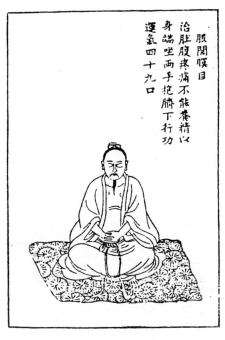

服閉暝目
治肚腹疼痛不能飲精以
身端坐兩手抱臍下行功
運氣四十九口

Figure 7

Song Xuanbai's method of healing indigestion (Fig. 8): Lie on the back and massage the abdomen up and down, while exhaling through mouth nine times. This serves to cure indigestion.

Qian Keng's method of healing lower back and leg pain (Fig. 9): Stand solidly, feet slightly apart. Make fists and bend forward until knuckles touch the ground. Then stand up and raise hands above the head. Close mouth and exhale slightly through nose three or four times. Repeat the movement several times.

Jie Yu's method of healing lower back pain (Fig. 10):

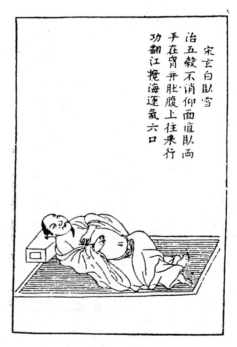

宋玄白臥雪
治五穀不消仰面直臥兩
手在胃并肚腹上往來行
功翻江捲海運氣六口

Figure 8

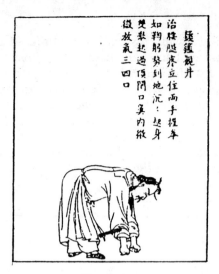

鐵鐘觀井
治膝腿疼立住兩手提拳
如鈎肩勢到地沉：起身
雙拳起過頂門口鼻內微
微放氣三四口

Figure 9

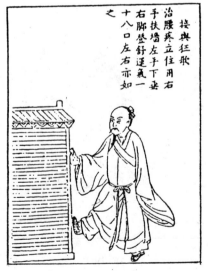

接與狂歌
治腰疼立住用右
手扶墙左手下垂
右脚登舒運氣一
十八口左右亦如
之

Figure 10

Stand facing a wall. Press palm of right hand against the wall, let the left hand hang naturally and place right foot against the wall. Then exhale slowly through mouth 18 times. Repeat this with left hand and foot on the wall. This exercise serves to heal lower back pain including strain of lumbar muscles, hyperplasia of bones and lumbago.

Zhong Li's method of healing lower back and leg pain (Fig. 11): Sit upright, rubbing hands together until

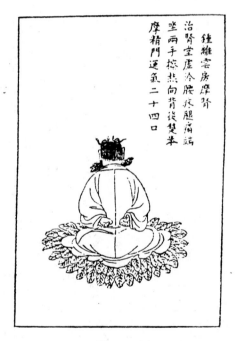

Figure 11

they are warm. Massage the lower back until its skin becomes warm, then tap at the waist with fists. Repeat many times. This exercise heals deficiency of the kidney, lower back and leg pain, coldness and pain at the waist, lumbago and strain of lumber muscles.

Liu Hai's method of healing aches and pains all over the body (Fig. 12): Stand with left foot forward. Clench fists at sides and exhale slowly through mouth 12 times. Do the same with right foot forward. Repeat several

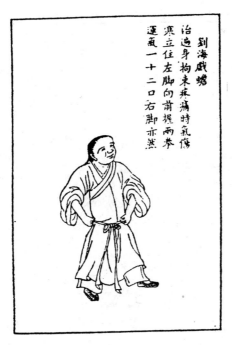

Figure 12

times. This serves to heal common cold and aches all over the body.

Imperial Brother-in-law Cao's method of healing paralysis (Fig. 13): Sit on bed with left foot brought nearly to the right thigh. Clench both hands into fists and raise them upward to the left of the body. Exhale through the mouth 24 times with the eyes straining to the right. Repeat several times, alternating positions and directions. This exercise heals paralysis. If a patient cannot do it on his own, someone should help move his

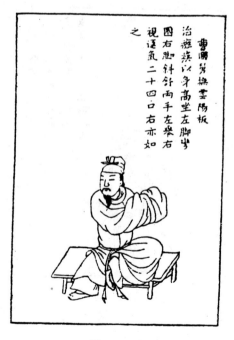

Figure 13

limbs.

Yu Zi's method of healing paralysis (Fig. 14): Point forward with the left hand in front of the body, with eyes looking to the right while exhaling through the mouth 24 times. Reverse positions and repeat the breathing exercise. A patient of paralysis can practise this exercise repeatedly with somebody else's assistance.

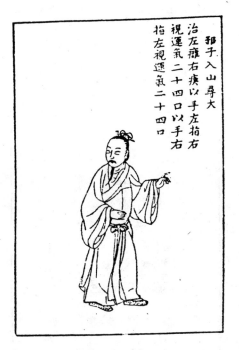

Figure 14

Shan Tu's method of healing nocturnal emission (Fig. 15): Sit on bed with feet stretched in front. Reach feet with hands and massage the balls of the feet while exhaling through mouth nine times. Repeat many times.

Chen Xiyi's method of healing sexual exhaustion (Fig. 16): With right hand as pillow, lie on the side on a bed. Press left leg on right leg. Massage abdomen with left hand and concentrate the mind at *dantian*. Inhale through the nose 32 times and direct *qi* into *dantian*. Repeat many times. This exercise serves to heal general debility caused by excessive sexual behaviour.

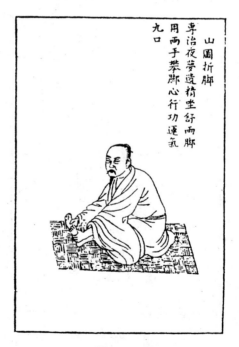

Figure 15

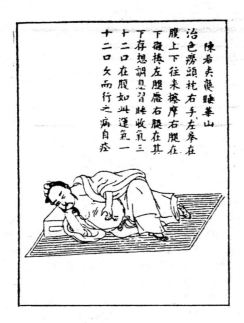

陳希夷龍蟄睡華山
治色勞頭枕右手,左拳在
腹上下往来撺摩右腿在
下微捲左腿展右腿在其
下存想調息習睡收氣三
十二口在腹如此運氣一
十二口久而行之病自痊

Figure 16

Quiescent *Qigong*

This *qigong* exercise includes three essential elements: adjusting the body (posture), regulating the breath (respiration) and regulating the mind (meditation).

Adjusting the body: A natural relaxed posture is the prerequisite for successful *qigong* breathing. Relaxation of the body can also induce mental relaxation and the posture itself also has curative effects. Common postures are seated, lying and standing. Seated and lying postures

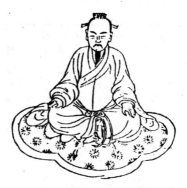

Figure 1

are most suitable for the elderly as they practise *qigong*.

Seated form: There are two seated postures. One is sitting with crossed legs on a bed (Fig. 1) and the other is sitting on a low, broad, level stool. The most popular posture is sitting on a square stool with feet flat on the ground, legs forward and feet shoulder-width apart. Sit with head upright, torso straight, shoulders low and loose, chest in, eyes slightly closed, mouth naturally shut and upper teeth set lightly against lower teeth, the tip of tongue naturally touching the upper palate, the hands resting in a relaxed manner on the legs or clasped lightly below the knees as depicted in the ancient *qigong* diagram (Fig. 2).

Lying form: One may lie on the back or on the side. It is more suitable for elderly people to lie on the side. In general, lie on the right side with right arm bent beside the body and right hand on pillow (Fig. 3). The left arm is extended naturally, hand on hip with palm downward. The right leg bends naturally and the left leg extends slightly. The eyes, mouth and tongue are posi-

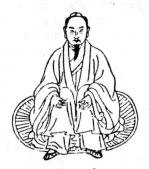

Figure 2

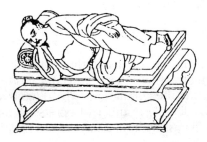

Figure 3

tioned as described for the seated postures.

Regulating breathing: This comes after adjusting the posture. Deep abdominal breathing is often used. When inhaling, the abdomen expands and when exhaling, it contracts. Breathing should become deeper and deeper until a rhythm of no more than eight to nine breaths per minute is achieved. It is necessary to relax and not exert oneself. Regulate the breathing to make it thin, deep, long, slow, steady, quiet and even.

Regulating the mind: While regulating the breath, fall into a tranquil mental state. Clear the mind of all thoughts and let it rest on *dantian*. This brings the experienced *qigong* practitioner into an ethereal state of warmth, lightness and tranquility. Anyone can achieve this state by persistent practice. If a beginner finds it difficult to concentrate his attention at *dantian* over a long time, he may imagine a ball with *dantian* as the centre. The ball either sparkles with a golden light or looks like a luminous emerald. One may develop all sorts of beautiful images to help concentrate the mind. It is also possible to concentrate the mind on the balls of the feet or on the toes.

Massage

Massage is one of the traditional Chinese methods for building the physique. It prevents and treats diseases by promoting the circulation of blood and *qi*. China has had a considerable number of books on massage from different dynasties, and today it has hospitals specializing in massage.

There are a great variety of massaging methods. Recommended here are massages to prevent wrinkles, to keep legs and knees fit and for propping the scrotum.

Massage face to prevent wrinkles: Ancient scholars on the art of healthy living held that rubbing the face preserves a youthful countenance. If one often massages the face, it will be ruddy, glossy and smooth-skinned with few wrinkles. This method is described in the book *Essentials for Spiritual and Physical Cultivation (Xing Ming*

Gui Zhi) written by Yin Zhenren, a Daoist recluse of the Ming Dynasty: "Often rub the face to warm it. Whenever one has leisure, he may massage the face. This makes it lustrous without wrinkles. Massage over a long period and one's countenance will always remain youthful."

In general, after getting up in early morning and before going to bed, rub hands until they are warm, then massage with palms from forehead down to chin and from the outer corners of eyes to the back of the ears. Be gentle and even in the movements. Massage 30 to 100 times every morning and evening. Unceasing practise enables the elderly to remain youthful in countenance.

Massage to keep legs and knees fit: Aging first begins at one's legs, the Chinese believe, so that massaging legs and knees can combat senility. Rubbing legs is beneficial to blood and lymphatic circulation in the lower limbs. Consequently it can prevent varicosity, orthostatic edema, and atrophy of lower extremities. Massaging knees can raise their temperature, promote the flexibility of the joints to facilitate movement and prevent arthritis of the knees.

Sit on bed or a stool (Fig. 1). Massage with both

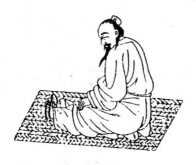

Figure 1

hands from thighs downward to the knees and the shin bones. Repeat ten times until the skin of the thighs and legs warms up. Or hold firmly the tops of the thighs near the hips and rub downward vigorously to the ankles, and then rub back to the tops of the thighs, thus rubbing up and down over 20 times until the skin of the legs and feet warms up. Press kneecaps firmly with the palms, first turning them inward more than 10 times, then turning them outward more than 10 times and then rubbing the knees with the palms until the skin warms up.

Massage around the scrotum (Fig. 2): This exercise is something of a secret treasure among ancient scholars on the art of healthy living. Among the common people it is known as the "iron crotch exercise." The key of the exercise, which has many varieties, is the stimulation of the testicles. Testicles secrete male hormone, which promotes and maintains the normal development and functioning of male accessory organs. Male hormones also play an important role in maintaining the body's health and prolonging life. The exercise is performed in the following steps:

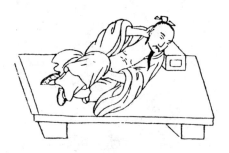

Figure 2

First, rub hands until they are warm. Lift the scrotum with one hand and put the little finger of the other hand slantwise near the pubes below the lower abdomen. Then rub with both hands the testes and penis vigorously upward about 100 times. Change hands and repeat. When first starting, rub gently and for fewer times. After some practise and conditioning, use more vigour and increase the massage strokes to several hundred.

Second, rub hands until they are warm, then rub testes and penis between the fingers with appropriate strength about 100 times.

Third, stretch testes in one hand and penis in the other vigorously three to five times.

Fourth, rub testes with fingers, alternating hands, then rub the lower abdomen dozens of times.

When doing this exercise, strength and duration should be increased gradually. The procedure should not cause pain or discomfort. But as the massaged parts are conditioned, work at it as vigorously as possible for several hundred times, giving sufficient testicle stimulus. Men who are impotent or suffer from premature ejaculation due to sexual decline and old men of general debility are best suited for this exercise. It does not suit young men because improper practice may easily lead to masturbation. It is suitable to perform this exercise under bed covers before rising and after retiring. Attention should be paid to cleanliness of the private parts. If they are afflicted with inflammation or eczema, it is better not to perform this exercise until these diseases have been cured.

At least one aged peasant, whose white hair is a delightful contrast to his youthful countenance, claims the secret of his good health and longevity lies precisely in performing this exercise. Gu Daifeng who wrote the book *Massage for Health Care* suffered from a severe disease because of overstudy when he was in middle age. He resorted to all sorts of treatment to no avail. His father taught him the exercise of propping the scrotum. Only by persistently practising this exercise did he succeed in eliminating diseases and prolonging life. He lived into his 90s, dying only a few years ago.

Teeth-Tapping Exercise

The exercise of tapping teeth and swallowing saliva has been mentioned earlier. The way to do it is as follows.

Early every morning, close the mouth lightly and tap molars together, then front teeth, then canine teeth, 36 times each. Then let the tongue tip touch the upper palate and blow up cheeks to rinse mouth. Swallow the accumulated saliva in three gulps.

This can strengthen teeth and prevent dental ailments. One who has persistently tapped his teeth for decades is now in his 60s with his whole set of teeth in place and in good condition. One person reported tapping his teeth together 200 times in the morning and again at night, curing periodontitis. As a folk saying instructs, "Tap teeth together 36 times in early morning and your teeth will not fall out when you are old."

Lick with the tongue around the inside of the mouth and rinse the mouth by circulating an air bubble to stretch cheeks and lips. This can stimulate the secretion of saliva which contains amylase, lysozyme and secretory antibody, helping to digest food, killing bacteria and viruses. Recent studies have shown the saliva gland can synthesize certain bioactive substances which act on the growth of blood sodium and blood sugar. Evidently, it was a sound scientific principle for ancient scholars on the art of healthy living to urge people to "prize saliva as gold."

Traditional Chinese Medicine

Medicine for Attaining a Tortoise's Long Life (*Gui Ling Ji*)

Origin: It was a secret court prescription used by Emperor Shi Zong of the Ming Dynasty and was formerly called "Lord Lao Zi's longevity pill." The court physician who prepared this medicine, a native of Taigu County, Shanxi Province, secretly took the prescription from the palace, starting the spread of this herbal preparation to ordinary people. Emperor Qian Long of the Qing Dynasty often took this medicine, as well as following other health practices, to become the longest-lived of recorded emperors.

Composition: Ginseng, pilose antler, sea horse, the fruit of Chinese wolfberry (*Lycium chinense*), sparrow's brain, dragonfly and 22 others.

Effective for: Dimmed vision, tinnitus, cerebrovascular sclerosis, chronic gastritis and especially male sexual decline. It strengthens the physique, benefits the brain, prevents and eliminates diseases, slows aging and prolongs life.

Forms of preparation: Powder or wine.

Producer: Shanxi Provincial Herbal Medicine Factory.

Male Treasire (*Nan Bao*)

Origin: Based on the theory that good health and

longevity depend on the vital energy of the kidney, researchers of Houma Herbal Medicine Factory of Shanxi Province analysed and sifted efficient prescriptions for the treatment of kidney deficiency and used precious herbs to prepare this medicine.

Composition: Kidneys of donkey and dog, sea horse, Dong'o glue made of donkey's skin, root of membraneous milkvetch (*Astragalus membranaceus*), the fruit of medicinal cornel (*Cornus officinalis*), ginseng, pilose antler and 23 others.

Effective for: Deficiency and decline of the vital energy of the kidneys, impotence and nocturnal emission; lumbago and leg pain; humidity and chill of the scrotum; listlessness, and poor appetite. This preparation is effective in nourishing the kidney, preventing premature aging, and promoting male sexual function.

Form of preparation: Capsules.

Producer: Houma Herbal Medicine Factory of Shanxi Province.

Precious Triple-Whip Pill (*Zhi Bao San Bian Wan*)

Origin: Yantai Pharmaceutical Factory of Shandong Province and Yanji Herbal Medicine Factory of Jilin Province jointly produce this medical preparation on the basis of popular anti-aging prescriptions.

Composition: Penises ("whips") of sika deer, fur seal and dog; sea horse; clam oil; ginseng, and 35 other herbal medicines.

Effective for: General weakness, premature aging, brain exhaustion, nocturnal emission, sexual decline, weakness of the heart, shortness of breath and tendencies to fatigue. This preparation will invigorate semen, nourish the kidneys, strengthen the physique and prolong life.

Forms of preparation: There are a series of products. Among them are "precious triple-whip essence" (*Zhi Bao San Bian Jing*), an oral solution produced by Yantai Pharmaceutical Factory of Shandong Province; "precious triple-whip pill" (*Zhi Bao San Bian Wan*) produced by Yantai Herbal Medicine Factory, and "multi-whip essence" (*Duo Bian Jing*), an oral solution manufactured by No. 2 Herbal Medicine Factory of Yanji City, Jilin Province.

Thorny Slender Acanthopanax Nutrient

Origin: Li Shizhen's *Compendium of Materia Medica* (*Ben Cao Gang Mu*) records examples of people taking thorny slender acanthopanax to prolong life, saying, "One has rather obtain a handful of slender acanthopanax than a cart of gold and jade." Ordinary people have used thorny slender acanthopanax to treat general weakness and various chronic diseases of the elderly.

Harbin No. 1 and No. 2 Herbal Medicine Factories of Heilongjiang Province manufacture thorny slender acanthopanax powders and slender acanthopanax essence respectively. These and the thorny slender acanthopanax tablets produced by the Kuancheng Pharmaceutical Factory of Hebei Province are all serial products of thorny slender acanthopanax nutrients. They produce similar effects.

Composition: Thorny slender acanthopanax (*Acanthopanax senticosus*), a medicinal herb similar to ginseng.

Effective for: Chronic diseases of weakness in the elderly, such as tracheitis, sexual decline, primary hypertension, neurasthenia, premature debility and premature aging. The preparation nourishes the kidneys, benefits the spleen, strengthens tendons and bones, benefits the brain and calms the mind, promotes circulation of *qi* and reduces phlegm. It is remarkable in slowing aging and enhancing abilities to adapt to environment.

Forms of preparation: Thorny slender acanthopanax nutrient is made in capsules. There are also soluble powders and tablets.

Youth Treasure (*Qing Chun Bao*)

Origin: Made of medicinal herbs according to a prescription of the Imperial Hospital of the Yongle Reign (1403-1424) in the Ming Dynasty.

Composition: Ginseng and many other medicinal herbs.

Effective for: Failing memory in the elderly, senile dementia, decline in resistance to disease, premature aging, weakness of the heart and coronary heart disease. This preparation can strengthen the physique, delay senility, benefit the brain, calm the mind, invigorate thinking, maintain vitality and vigour, strengthen immunity, promote resistance to disease, improve nutrition of cardiac muscle and postpone the formation and development of coronary heart disease.

Forms of preparation: In both liquid and tablet forms.

Producer: Hangzhou No. 2 Herbal Medicine Factory.

Life-Prolonging Tea (*Yi Shou Cha*)

Origin: Produced from local teas and medicinal herbs by Yuhuan County Drink and Food Factory of Zhejiang Province.

Effective for: Obesity, foul breath and erosion of lips and tongue caused by hypertension, hyperlipemia, arteriosclerosis and accumulations of fat. Also effective on tachycardia. The preparation reduces fat, facilitates bowel movement, digests food, clears internal heat, reduces weight and increases the secretion and flow of urine.

Forms of preparation and usage: Herbal tea slices in 50 g nylon bag or 80 g metal box; 2-3 g each time, steeped in boiling water for drinking, once or twice daily.

Chinese Life-Preserving Wine (*Yang Sheng Jiu*)

Origin: This wine dates back to the Tang Dynasty. Legend has it that Tang Emperor Xuan Zong became infatuated with his favourite concubine, Lady Yang, growing sallow, emaciated and listless. Then an imperial physician said to the emperor: "When I toured east to Shangluo, I heard of an old man in his 140s on Funiu Hill. He has 54 sons and daughters. His eldest son is 123 years old and his youngest daughter only two years old."

The astonished emperor immediately sent for the old man. The Grandpa, with black hair and youthful countenance, entered the palace with vigorous strides, looking as if he were still in the prime of life. The emperor asked him about the key to his longevity. Grandpa told him, "I've often drunk a fine wine brewed with the essence of a hundred flowers and countless medicines and the water of a five-source spring." He presented the wine he had brought with him to the emperor. After drinking the wine, Emperor Xuan Zong's spirit refreshed and his health recovered. The prescription was rediscovered in the annals of Xixia County in 1949.

Effective for: Male sexual decline, impotence, premature aging, neurasthenia, soreness and fatigue of the spine and lower back, male and female sterility and rheumatic arthritis. It promotes blood circulation, regulates the mechanism of the whole body, invigorates the spirit, nourishes the blood, preserves black hair and youthful countenance and prolongs life.

Producer: Xixia County Fruit Wine Factory of Henan Province.

Dongtian Chinese Gooseberry Wine

Origin: Dongtian Chinese Gooseberry (*Actinidia chinensis*) Wine has been brewed for 1,200 years with the berry as its main ingredient, by Daoist priests of Qingcheng Mountain in Guanxian County, Sichuan Province. It is full of nutrition, having unusually rich aroma and a sweet flavour with a sour tinge. Mellow and moistening, it refreshes the mind and soothes the spleen.

Effective for: Indigestion, poor appetite, hypertension, hemiplegia, skin diseases, insomnia and the formation of stones in the urinary system. Drinking the wine over a long period turns one's white hair black and prolongs one's life span.

Producer: The Daoist temple on Qingcheng Mountain in Guanxian County, Sichuan Province.

Shaolin Medicinal Wine

Origin: Its prescription was worked out by Henan College of Traditional Chinese Medicine with the directions of monk physicians and herb growers in Shaolin Monastery, Henan Province.

Shaolin Medicinal Wine has two varieties, "Bodhidharma Strength-Increasing Wine" and "Buddhist Monk Secret Wine." The former is dark brown and has a rich herbal aroma. It promotes and invigorates blood circulation, reduces phlegm, nourishes vital energy and increases strength. It helps to heal injuries from falls, fractures, contusions and strains, rheumatism, rheumatoid arthritis and senile cardiovascular diseases. "Buddhist Monk Secret Wine" is crystal-clear, tonic and nourishing. It slows aging and prolongs life.

Producer: Linhe Wine Factory of Henan Province.

Food Therapy

Food therapy for longevity provides nourishing, health-building foods with tonic medicines of herbal and animal origin. Turning bitter medicine into delicious dishes, such food therapy is mild in nature and without toxic or other unfavourable side effect. It can both appease hunger and prevent diseases and can be taken over a long period in ordinary circumstances. For healthy people it can maintain health, slow aging and prevent diseases. For people of weak constitution it can strengthen the physique, slow senility and increase the resistance to disease, hence building health and prolonging life. There are a great number of records and legends about longevity recipes in ancient Chinese books and among the common people. Following are a few carefully selected ones.

Chinese Wolfberry Porridge

Method of cooking: Thirty g of Chinese wolfberry and 60 g of round-grained rice, boiled together into porridge.

Function: Taken mornings and evenings, it combats senility, strengthens the physique and prolongs life.

Shen Nong's Materia Medica records: "Taking Chinese wolfberry over a long time strengthens tendons and bones and makes one lithe and youthful." Zhen Quan, a famous centenarian physician in the Tang Dynasty, wrote in his *On the Nature of Herbs* (*Yao Xing Ben Cao*):

"Chinese wolfberry improves vision, tranquilizes the mind and makes people live long." Modern studies show that Chinese wolfberry improves the immune function of the human body.

Walnut Porridge

Method of cooking: Ten to fifteen chopped walnuts boiled with 60 g of round-grained rice into porridge.

Function: Taken mornings and evenings, it prevents and cures pulmonary tuberculosis, chronic tracheitis, constipation and calculus of the urinary system of the elderly. Taken over a long time, it benefits the brain and prevents senile dementia.

Compendium of Materia Medica (*Ben Cao Gang Mu*) records: "Eating walnuts can strengthen tendons and bones, moisten the skin and keep the hair black, and nourish blood and marrow." Modern studies show that walnut contains various amino acids and therefore can provide protein needed by the human body, promote the growth of brain cells and improve the function of the cerebra. Consequently it delays senility.

Knotweed Porridge

Method of cooking: First boil 30 to 60 g of prepared knotweed (tuber of the multiflower knotweed) into a thick decoction in an earthen pot and remove the dregs. Then boil the decoction with 60 g of round-grained rice, three large red dates and crystal sugar into porridge.

Function: Eaten morning and evening, it nourishes the blood, strengthens the physique, delays senility, treating dizziness, tinnitus, premature aging, anaemia, neurasthenia, hyperlipemia, vascular sclerosis and constipation.

Knotweed is a widely known anti-senility medicine in China, the subject of many legends. *Compendium of*

Materia Medica told of a man named He Tianer of Xingtai, Hebei, who by taking knotweed reached the age of 130. His son followed suit and also became a centenarian. Ming Emperor Shi Zong, as a legend goes, was cured of sterility by a prescription with knotweed as its main ingredient.

Modern studies show that knotweed contains lecithin, which promotes the function of the nervous system and the heart. It can reduce blood fat and prevent arteriosclerosis and senile hyperlipemia. It can improve the immune system and delay the aging of the nerves and blood vessels.

Lean Pork Steamed with Sealwort (*Polygonatum sibiricum*)

Method of cooking: Wash 50 g of sealwort and 200 g of lean pork. Cut both into slivers 3 cm long and 1.5 cm wide. Put them in an earthen pot and add water, scallions, ginger, salt and cooking wine. Steam them until well done. Add monosodium glutamate when serving. The sealwort can be eaten along with the pork.

Function: It treats emaciation, poor appetite, atrophic gastritis, coronary heart disease and insomnia. It nourishes the heart and spleen, improves the immunity function and delays aging.

Eight-Treasure Chicken Soup

Method of cooking: Combine these Chinese herbs, 10 g each of dangshen (*Codonopsis pilosula*), fuling (*Poris cocos*), the rhizome of large-headed atractylodes and root of herbaceous peony; 15 g each of prepared rhizome of rehmannia (*Rehmannia glutinosa*) and Chinese angelica; 5 g of rhizome of chuanxiong (*Ligusticum wallichii*) and 6 g of roast liquorice root. Put the herbs in a firmly tied gauze bag and soak the bag in water for a short while. Wash a fat hen (about one kilo), 1,500 g of pork and 1,500 g of pig bones pound into pieces. Wash and slice 40 g of fresh ginger, wash 100 g of scallions and tie them into a small sheaf. After preparing these ingredients, put chicken meat, pork, bones and the bag of medicinal herbs into the pot, add water to cover them and boil on high heat. Skim the scum, add ginger and scallions and stew on gentle fire until chicken and pork are well-done. Finally remove the medicinal bag, ginger and scallions from the soup. Take out chicken and pork and cut them into slivers. Put them in a bowl, pour in strained hot soup and add monosodium glutamate and salt to make the dish ready for serving.

Function: It treats general debility, poor immunity function and various chronic ailments in the elderly. It reinforces the physique, nourishes the blood and vital energy, increases physical strength, and delays senility.

Multi-Herb Nourishing Soup

Method of cooking: Take 10 g each of dangshen, membranous milkvetch, the rhizome of large-headed atractylodes and fuling; 15 g each of prepared rhizome of rehmannia and Chinese angelica; 3 g of Chinese cassia tree; 12 g of the root of herbaceous peony, and 6 g each of the rhizome of chuanxiong and liquorice root. Wash and put them into a gauze bag and close firmly. Put 50 g of cuttlefish, 500 g of pork, 50 g of pig stomach and pig bones pounded into pieces into a pot with the medicinal bag. Add water, 30 g of ginger, scallions, cooking wine, Chinese prickly ash and salt. First bring these to a boil on high heat, then stew on gentle heat. When the pork is well-done, remove from heat, take out the medicinal bag, eat the pork and drink the soup. It should be taken morning and evening.

Function: It can be taken frequently, especially in winter, by elderly individuals who are frail after long illnesses or suffer from vital energy and blood deficiency, weakness of the limbs, listlessness, hypotension, anaemia or cancer.

Whole Duck Steamed with Chinese Caterpillar Fungus

Method of cooking: Collect 10 g of Chinese caterpillar fungus, an old drake and cooking wine, ginger, white scallion stalks, pepper and salt. First, parboil the drake in boiling water and spread it to cool in the air. Clean Chinese caterpillar fungus with warm water, cut ginger and scallion into slices. Then split the drake open from the head and along the neck, stuff eight to ten Chinese caterpillar fungi into its head, tie it firmly with cotton thread and sew the remaining Chinese caterpillar fungus, ginger and scallion stalk into the body cavity. Put all these into a jar and fill with clear soup stock. Flavour with salt, pepper and cooking wine. Cover the jar with wet cotton paper and steam in a closed steamer for two hours. Remove cotton paper and pick out the ginger, scallion stalk and add monosodium glutamate. It is ready to serve.

Function: It treats chronic coughing and shortness of breath, chronic tracheitis, pulmonary emphysema and lung cancer. It strengthens the physique, moistens the lungs, allays coughing and improves the immunity function.

Carp Steamed with the Tuber of Elevated Gastrodia

Method of cooking: Assemble 15 g of the tuber of natural elevated gastrodia, 3 g of the rhizoma of chuanxiong (*Ligusticum wallichii*) and 9 g of fuling (*Poris cocos*), a fresh carp (about 500 to 1,000 g), soy sauce, cooking wine, sugar, monosodium glutamate, pepper, single-headed garlic, sesame oil, scallions, ginger, and liquid bean starch. Remove scales, gill and internal organs from the carp. Wash and put it on a platter. Cut chuanxiong and fuling into large slices and soak them in water from the second washing of rice and soak the tuber of elevated gastrodia for four to six hours in the rice wash water in which chuanxiong and fuling have been soaked. Scoop up the tuber of elevated gastrodia and put it on rice, steaming both until well-done. Slice the gastrodia and place these slices in the fish head and belly. Add scallion, garlic and ginger and water. Steam in a closed steamer for about 30 minutes. When the fish is well-steamed, remove scallions and ginger. Then heat liquid bean starch, clear soup stock, sugar, salt, monosodium glutamate, pepper and sesame oil into a thick sauce and put it on the gastrodia carp for serving.

Function: It prevents and treats neurasthenia, hypertension, dizziness, numbness of the limbs, unfavourable after-effects of stroke and other heart and brain vascular diseases. It tranquilizes the mind and nourishes the brain.

Eel Broth with Chinese Angelica and Dangshen

Method of cooking: Select 15 g of top-quality Chinese angelica and dangshen each and 500 g of fresh eels. Collect cooking wine, scallions, ginger, garlic, monosodium glutamate and soy sauce. Cut open the eels, remove the internal organs, heads, tails and bones and cut them into shreds. Put dangshen and Chinese angelica into a gauze bag and tie its opening. Put eel shreds into a pot, add cooking wine, scallions, garlic, ginger, salt, water and the medicinal bag. Bring the pot to a boil over high heat, skim the scum and stew it on gentle heat for about an hour. Remove the medicinal bag and add monosodium glutamate. The soup is ready to serve.

Function: It treats general weakness after long illness, sallowness and emaciation, general lassitude, and anaemia. It nourishes the blood and vital energy.

Shrimp, Sea Horse and Young Chicken

Method of cooking: Assemble 15 g of shrimp meat, 10 g of sea horse, a young male chicken, cooking wine, monosodium glutamate, salt, ginger, scallions, liquid bean starch and clear soup. Kill the chicken, remove its feathers and internal organs and wash it clean. Clean sea horse and shrimp meat in warm water and soak them in water for 10 minutes. Scoop them up and scatter them over the chicken on a platter, adding ginger, scallions and clear soup. Steam in a closed steamer until very well-done. Remove meat, scallions and ginger. Add monosodium glutamate to the soup and stir in liquid bean starch for a thick sauce to pour over the meat for serving.

Function: It treats sexual decline, impotence, premature ejaculation and sterility. It promotes secretions of the sexual gland and prevents its atrophy.

Double-Whip Soup

Collect 10 g each of Chinese wolfberry, the seeds of Chinese dodder, and saline cistanche (*Cistanche salsa*); 100 g of ox penis, 30 g of dog penis, 100 g of mutton, 50 g of hen meat, Chinese prickly ash, old ginger, cooking wine, gourmet powder, lard and salt. First, soak ox penis in water to enlarge it. Remove the superficial skin, split into two halves along the urinary duct, scrub with fresh water and soak in cold water for 30 minutes. Stir-fry the dog penis with oily sand until it becomes crisp, soak in warm water for about 30 minutes and brush and clean thoroughly. Wash the mutton and parboil in a pot of boiling water to remove blood water, cool and wash in cold water. Then put ox penis, dog penis and mutton into a pot, cover with water, bring to a boil and skim the scum. Put Chinese prickly ash, old ginger, cooking wine and hen meat into the pot. Again bring to a boil, then stew on low heat. When it is sixty percent done, filter off with clean white cloth the Chinese prickly ash and old ginger. Put the pot again on the stove, place a gauze bag containing the seeds of Chinese dodder, saline cistanche and Chinese wolfberry into the soup and continue stewing until the penises are very well done. Remove the medicinal bag. Add monosodium glutamate, salt and lard to the remaining soup to make it ready to serve.

Function: It treats general debility and sexual decline of the aged, male impotence, seminal emission, premature ejaculation and chronic prostatitis. It nourishes the kidneys, invigorates the vital energy and improves sexual function.

Prevention and Self-Treatment of Common Old-Age Diseases

Common Cold

Symptoms: Headache, pains all over the body, chills, a running and stuffy nose and cough.

Prevention: Common cold can endanger the lives of old people with weak constitutions. Moreover, "a hundred diseases start from the common cold." So the elderly should take positive measures for prevention described here:

1. Self massaging. After getting up in the morning, or before going out, first pinch and press *yingxiang* point (near the two sides of the nostrils) with fingers for one to three minutes or rub both sides of the nose bridge with forefingers until they are warm. Then press *renzhong* point (the depression between the nose and the upper lip) dozens of times. This energizes the immunity faculty of the body to resist effects of climatic fluctuations.

2. For those with weak constitutions and vulnerability to colds, take decoctions boiled with 50 g of membraneous milkvetch, or meat stewed with this medicinal herb, or frequently eat multi-herb nourishing soup (see recipe in the previous section on food therapy). This can improve the immunity faculty and reduce occurrences of the common cold.

Treatment:

1. For severe symptoms of chills, aches all over the body, no thirst and much clear urine, boil several slices of ginger and brown sugar in water until a fairly strong liquid results. Drink while steaming hot, lie down covered with a quilt until there is slight perspiration.

2. If the patient has marked symptoms of fever, sore throat, thirst and infrequent yellow urination, he may take *Yin Qiao Jie Du Pian* (detoxicating tablets prepared from honeysuckle and weeping forsythia) and *Ling Qiao Jie Du Pian* (tablets containing antelope's horn and weeping forsythia), or dyers woad powder.

If the ailment has not been alleviated after being treated with the above-mentioned methods for two days, the patient should see a doctor for diagnosis and treatment.

Chronic Tracheitis

Attacks of chronic tracheitis usually come in winter and the patient may continue coughing for more than three months. Often the patient will have a case history of three to five years, or even decades of this annual affliction. Its main symptoms are coughing, particularly in mornings and evenings, plenty of phlegm and shortness of breath, sometimes complications of asthma occur and the condition is often induced or aggravated by a common cold.

Prevention: Senile chronic tracheitis easily develops into emphysema and pulmonary heart disease so the patient should prevent, if possible, and treat early when it occurs.

1. Methods used to prevent common cold can prevent acute attacks of chronic tracheitis.

2. Abstain from smoking.

3. Practise *qigong* or *taijiquan* to build the physique.

Treatment: There are many methods and medicines, but few can cure chronic tracheitis radically. Therefore, stress is laid on its prevention.

1. During acute attacks of chronic tracheitis, take *Qing Fei Yi Huo Hua Tan Wan* (pills for clearing the lungs, alleviating the febrile symptoms and reducing phlegm) and *Zhu Li Da Tan Wan* (pills containing extracts from roast bamboo stalks for eliminating phlegm) and *Ling Qiao Jie Du Wan* (detoxicating pills made from antelope's horn and weeping forsythia).

2. In ordinary times the patient may take such medical preparations as *Jin Long Dan Pian* (herba conyzae tablets) of Sichuan Province, *Re Shen Pian* (radix physochlainae tablets) of Shaanxi Province, *Mu Jing Wan* (*Vitex negundo* pills) of Fujian Province and *Zhao Shan Bai* (*Rhododendron micranthum* tablets) of Beijing. All these medicines produce good effects for alleviating cough and asthma and eliminating phlegm.

3. Those with weak constitutions may take in ordinary times four-nut egg porridge. Put one part gingko and sweet almond and two parts walnut and peanut together to grind into powder. Boil 20 g of this, mix with an egg in a small bowl and drink early every morning for six months, starting in early autumn before tracheitis attacks and continuing to the next spring.

4. The patient can often take food therapy, "duck steamed with Chinese caterpillar fungus." It has fairly good effect on the elderly who are emaciated and suffer long from coughing and shortness of breath. Those who gasp and perspire with every movement and often suffer from common colds can frequently take food therapy "multi-herb nourishing soup" to increase resist-

ance to diseases and prevent common cold from inducing tracheitis.

Coronary Heart Disease

Coronary heart disease is common among the elderly, especially   intellectuals. Its main symptoms are angina pectoris, arrhythmia and myocardial infarction.

Angina pectoris: This is caused by the narrowing and cramping of coronary arteries and an inadequate supply of oxygen for cardiac muscles. During an attack there are various signs. Some patients feel restrictions in the chest as if breathing were going to stop; some suffer from faint pains in the cardiac area of the chest; some feel as if a slab of stone weighed heavily on the chest; some feel pain in the heart as if something were grabbing, clutching or pulling at it; some feel smarting as if being pricked by many needles. The area of pain is located in the front cardiac area at left chest or under the chest bone or in the centre of the heart. The pain can radiate to shoulders, more severely on left shoulder and downwards to left arm and to left elbow and the ulna of left hand, and can also radiate to the throat and neck, lasting several seconds or minutes. It may occur when overfatigued, angry, taking a meal, when cold, while smoking or after drinking alcohol.

Myocardial infarction: This is caused by the necrosis of cardiac muscle due to the complete obstruction of coronary arteries. There are often signs of angina pectoris. It may be followed immediately by shock, lowered blood pressure, cold perspiration, blue and cold finger and toe nails, dizziness and even loss of consciousness. Sometimes sudden deaths occur, caused by myocardial infarction when the patient suddenly screams and dies.

Prevention: Diagnosis of a coronary disease requires

a physician but its prevention relies on the individual.

1. Traditional Chinese exercises are very effective in preventing cardiovascular diseases. Choose one or two kinds and persistently practise according to individual preference.

2. Reduce weight. In the main, rely on vegetarian foods, especially plenty of garlic, turnips and celery. This serves both for prevention and treatment.

3. Abstain from smoking and drink little alcohol. Smoking can stimulate cardiac blood vessels, causing damage, aggravating oxygen deficiencies of the cardiac muscles and inducing an attack of coronary disease. Drinking large quantities of alcohol over a long period will accelerate the development of coronary disease.

4. Prevent and treat related diseases. Coronary disease patients often suffer simultaneously from hypertension, diabetes and arteriosclerosis. These ailments often hasten each other and aggravate conditions.

5. Always remaining happy and keeping oneself warm against cold are also important preventive measures.

Treatment:

1. During attacks of angina pectoris the patient can take *Guan Xin Su He Pian* (tablets containing musk), *She Xiang Bao Xin Wan* (musk heart-preserving pills) and *She Xiang Tong Qi Wu Ji* (a musk-containing resuscitating aerosol).

2. In ordinary times the patiant may take *Dan Sheng Shu Xin Pian* (heart-relieving tablets containing the root of red-rooted salvia) of Shanghai.

3. When myocardial infarction occurs, summon a physician at once for emergency treatment. Before his arrival the patient may be pressed and rubbed at *ren-*

zhong (the depression between nose and upper lip) and *neiguan*. This allays pain, raises blood pressure and prevents shock.

4. Food therapy. If the patient suffers from arrhythmia, he may drink solutions from 30 g of the root of old tea bush boiled in water for auxiliary treatment, once every day until the heartbeat rhythm becomes regular.

Bean curd cooked with edible black fungus (*Auricularia auricula*) helps prevent and treat attacks of angina pectoris for coronary patients. Boil 60 g of bean curd and 15 g of black edible fungus with scallions and garlic. Eat the dish once every day or every other day. It will alleviate atherosclerosis.

Eating garlic and scallions frequently can reduce blood fat and dissipate blood clots. This reduces the attacks of angina pectoris and prevents myocardial infarction.

Boil 30 g of barley root hair with water as a daily drink. This alleviates angina pectoris for coronary patients.

Hypertension

As people reach 40 their chances of developing hypertension begin to increase each year. At the age of 65 and above, about 15 percent will suffer this affliction. A larger proportion of the overweight are afflicted with hypertension as their systolic pressures rise above 160 (mm Hg) and their diastolic pressures above 95 (mm Hg). Main clinical symptoms are dizziness, headache, lack of energy, insomnia, irritation and palpitations. In late stages the heart, brain or kidneys may be damaged. Heart damage brings about hypertensive heart diseases; brain damage causes apoplexy and kidney damage causes nephritis and uraemia.

Prevention: Methods for the prevention of coronary heart disease can also be applied to hypertension. Besides, hypertensives must pay special attention to diet and devote themselves to a low salt diet, a limit of about five grams of salt daily. Salt constricts blood vessels and causes water and sodium retention, resulting in or aggravating hypertension. It suits the hypertensives to eat foods high in protein such as fish and soy bean products. This can maintain elasticity of arteries and prevent hypertension.

Persist in practising *qigong*. Maintain optimistism and avoid mental traumatic experiences.

Treatment:

1. Food therapy: The patient can choose any of the following recipes according to individual conditions.

Frequently eat black edible fungus cooked with scallions and garlic. This can delay the formation of blood clots and reduce the occurrence of arteriosclerosis.

Soak peanuts in vinegar for a week. Eat 10 peanuts morning and evening. This softens blood vessels and reduces blood pressure.

Mix evenly 60 g of green bean flour and 120 g of pig gall juice, dry the mixture in the sun and grind it into fine powder. Three-gram doses should be taken three times a day. This can lower blood pressure.

Dry edible sea weeds in the sun and grind them into fine powder. Six g daily, divided into three doses, for one to three months. Edible sea weeds may also be stewed or steamed and eaten at meals. This can reduce blood pressure, prevent and treat cancer of the digestive tract.

Eat at least three apples each day after meals. This can lower blood pressure.

2. The patient can choose one of the following herbal preparations. *Nao Li Qing*, with chrysanthemum as its main ingredient, lowers blood pressure and sobers the brain; *Luo Bu Ma Pian*, compound bluish dogbane (*Apocynum venetum*) tablets; *Xin Jiang Ya Pian*, new-type tablets for reducing blood pressure, with *Uncaria rhynchophylla* and selfheal (*Prunella vulgaris*) as main ingredients; *Yu Feng Ning Xin Pian*, tablets with the root of kudzuvine as its main ingredient.

3. Rub the balls of the feet hundreds of times morning and evening to conduct the blood downwards.

Apply medicinal herb medicinal evodia to point *yongquan*. Grind the herb into fine powder, mix it with vinegar, apply the paste and cover with adhesive paster. Change dressings daily.

Wash feet with hot water every evening, washing upwards to the knees. Steep feet in hot water for more than half an hour.

Wash 10 g of sweet chrysanthemum leaves in clear water and steep them in a five-pound thermos flask to be taken as a daily drink, one flask per day.

Hypotension

People who suffer from hypotension have symptoms of drowsiness, dizziness, headache, insomnia, memory loss, inability to concentrate, fatigue or oppressive pain in the front cardiac area. With low blood pressure, slow blood flow increases coagulation of blood, making a patient susceptible to complications from the formation of blood clots, such as cerebral thrombus and myocardial infarction.

Prevention: Hypotension in old age is often related to weak constitution. So the patient should try to improve his general conditions.

1. It is necessary to treat the primary diseases contributing to hypotension, such as gastritis or ulcers. Persons of weak constitution may take tonic, nourishing medicines in ordinary times.

2. Patients of advanced years should move slowly in standing up, thus preventing orthostatic hypotension, and should avoid standing for long periods.

Treatment:

1. Take one of the following: ginseng and milkvetch essence of Jilin Province; ginseng and deer's antler tablet of Shanghai; *Qiong Jiang*, a tonic wine of Beijing with ginseng as its main ingredient.

2. If the patient is emaciated and has chills, he may put 0.3 g of deer's antler powder with an egg and steam them. Take a steamed deer antler egg early every morning for 15 to 30 days. It is unsuitable for elderly people to take this mixture over too long a period, or else it causes obesity and even hypertension.

3. Hypotensives may take food therapy such as "eight-treasure chicken soup," "multi-herb nourishing soup" and "angelica-ginseng eel broth" made from recipes in the food therapy section.

Apoplexy (Stroke)

Apoplexy, a common, critical disease of the elderly, has two types: blood-deficient and haemorrhagic. The former is mainly caused by the formation of blood clots in the brain resulting in hemiplegia. Haemorrhagic apoplexy comes violently and suddenly. The patient suddenly faints and becomes unconscious, with firmly locked jaws and convulsions of the limbs. Death may be immediate.

Prevention: Mortality in apoplexy is very high. It often comes too quickly to be treated or treatment is ineffective, making it of greatest importance to take preventive measures. As apoplexy in the elderly is mostly caused by hypertension and cerebral arteriosclerosis, those who suffer from these diseases should be especially careful.

1. Maintain a stable, composed frame of mind, a leisurely and rhythmic life pattern, and avoid mental stress and flashes of anger.

2. When the patient finds balance difficult and walks unsteadily, he should use a walking stick to avoid falling. He should move slowly when sitting down or standing up. Always move slowly.

3. Avoid stimulants such as smoking, alcohol, strong tea, strong coffee or cocoa. In ordinary times practise quiescent *qigong* persistently as a preventive measure.

Treatment: Treatment relies mainly on physicians. During an acute attack the following measures should be adopted before the physician's arrival.

1. Do not move the patient unless it is absolutely necessary. Let him lie flat on the back quietly. If the patient has fainted, put his head on a pillow with the chin slightly up. If he has vomited, it is better for him to lie on the side to prevent matter from entering the trachea to cause suffocation or pneumonia. Avoid movement of or by the patient, for such movement is likely to aggravate a cerebral haemorrhage. Quick professional medical care on the spot is crucial for avoiding death and reducing unfavourable after-effects.

2. Maintain smooth respiratory flow. Loosen the patient's collar, remove dentures and sheath an empty syringe with a rubber tube to suck phlegm from the throat.

3. If the patient moves restlessly or is convulsive, be

careful to prevent him from falling and hurting himself. If his jaws are locked and his limbs stiff, needle *renzhong* and the tips of ten fingers until they bleed. If his mouth gapes, hands are outstretched and he shows incontinence of feces and urine, press *renzhong* at once, and forcefully feed him ginseng essence and *Sheng Mai Ye* (a pulse recovering herbal liquid containing dwarf lily-turf and Chinese magnoliavine).

4. Hemiplegia and aphasia, the after-effects of apoplexy, can be treated with acupuncture and massage.

Chronic Gastritis

The elderly people who suffer from chronic atrophic gastritis, gastritis caused by the reverse flow of bile, or antrum gastritis can resort to herbal therapy. Chronic gastritis has symptoms of irregular, repeated stomach pains and indigestion.

Prevention: Without a doubt, chronic gastritis can be prevented if one takes proper care in one's daily life.

1. Mental tension and an improper balance between work and rest are important causes of chronic gastritis. Therefore, to be forthright and optimistic, to avoid mental depression and pay attention to a strict regimen and appropriate scheduling of work and rest are important measures for preventing chronic gastritis.

2. Both tobacco and alcohol can damage the mucous membrane of the stomach and lead to chronic gastritis, thus the necessity to abstain from smoking and strong drink. Some medicines such as aspirin, phenylbutazone, prednisone and erythromycin stimulate the stomach's mucous membrane and cause chronic gastritis, so they should be avoided as much as possible.

3. Intemperance in food and drink is the main cause of chronic gastritis. One should avoid eating and drink-

ing too much at meals and avoid food that tastes too sour, too peppery, too hot, too cold or too hard. It is especially essential to eat consistent amounts at regular time.

Treatment: Gastritis is not difficult to remedy but relapses easily occur.

1. If the patient has a low level of gastric acid, he may take hawthorn tablets or *Hericium erinaceus* tablets.

2. If stomach pains result when one feels cold or takes cold food or drink, he may take *Xiang Sha Liu Jun Zi Wan* or *Xiang Sha Yang Wei Wan*, pills with dang-shen and the rhizome of large-headed atractylodes as main ingredients.

3. Massage with left and right hands in turn around the navel for 30 to 100 times. Or press with three fingers slowly but vigorously at any point on the abdomen, pressing to a maximum depth before releasing slowly. Press the abdomen at each point for three to five times, progressing from upper abdomen to lower abdomen.

4. Food therapy: Boil the root of sorghum as a drink to treat gastric pains from feeling physically cold or from eating cold foods. Boil roots of three red sorghum plants with water into a daily drink.

Cholecystitis and Gallstone

Cholecystitis and gallstone (cholelithiasis) are common diseases of the aged. Autopsy has shown that 25 percent of people above the age of 60 and about 50 percent of those above the age of 70 have gallstones. As the walls of biliary ducts in the elderly thicken and become less elastic, inhibiting smooth flow of gall fluids, they stagnate in the bile-cyst, irritating its mucous membrane and causing inflammation. Moreover, it builds free bilirubin and cholesterol deposits which become gallstones. Besides, old people have reduced levels of gastric acid, making them susceptible to the bacterial infections which lead to cholecystitis.

Cholecystitis in the elderly often flares into acute attacks on chronic sufferers when triggered by the eating of eggs or greasy food or after a very heavy meal. Symptoms include pain in the upper right abdomen that may reach the right shoulder and right lower back, accompanied by nausea, vomiting, chills and fever. Some have symptoms of severe poisoning such as trembling and high fever. If a gallstone obstructs the bile duct, angina may occur, with a bloated and heavy feeling in the upper right abdomen and sometimes even jaundice (when face, eyes and the skin all over the body become yellowish.)

Cholelithiasis is often the outcome of chronic cholecystitis and gallstones often cause acute attacks of cholecystitis. Each is the cause and effect of the other.

Senile cholecystitis easily leads to acute pancreatitis, especially after a very full meal of greasy food or the drinking of alcoholic beverages. If acute upper abdominal pain suddenly occurs, a first thought should be for the possibility of acute pancreatitis. This can easily endanger life, so the patient should be taken to a hospital at once.

Prevention:

1. Obesity brings susceptibility to the disease. So, first of all, one should avoid becoming overweight.

2. Lifetime diet attention is important. It is unsuitable to eat food that is too greasy. Although vegetable oil is beneficial to excretion of gall fluids, it is not suitable when ingested in too large quantities. In particular, vegetable oil that has been stored too long or has been

used to fry other food easily oxidizes in the body and transforms itself into ester peroxidate, a carcinogenic substance.

3. Practising *taijiquan* and massage is beneficial to the excretion of gall fluids.

Treatment: Patients with cholecystitis can take medicines and a patient with a large gallstone should seek surgery to remove it.

1. Take medical preparations orally. *Li Dan Pian* (gall-benefitting tablets) and limonene capsules have good effects on cholecystitis. Centenarian physician Luo Mingshan of Sichuan Province has a secret prescription *Bai Cao Dan* (multi-herb pills) that treats cholecystitis and gallstones (within one cubic centimetre) effectively. In ordinary times the patient can also steep hemsley loosestrife of Sichuan Province in water as a daily drink.

2. The patient should be taken to hospital during acute attacks of cholecystitis with symptoms of general poisoning such as chills, trembling and high fever, and for gallstones bigger than one cubic centimetre.

3. As auxiliary treatment the patient of acute cholecystitis can take dandelion porridge. Gather 90 g of fresh dandelion (or 60 g if dry), wash and cut into pieces. Boil into a solution and remove the dregs. Add 50 g of round-grained rice and boil into a thin porridge. Eat three to five times a day for three to five days.

Senile Habitual Constipation

Old people often suffer chronically from constipation, accompanied by many related disorders such as irritation, insomnia, dizziness, fatigue, abdominal distension and pain, and poor appetite. This occurs mainly because their intestine muscles become atrophic, slowing peristalsis and losing the strength to excrete feces.

Hence, feces stay too long in the body and become hardened.

Prevention:

1. In ordinary times eat plenty of green-leaf vegetables. Especially good are potatoes and sweet potatoes because they contain a lot of cellulose and can strengthen the peristalsis of the intestines and facilitate bowel movement.

2. It is best to have a bowel movement regularly every morning after getting up or after breakfast. Go to the toilet at a fixed time each day whether the urge for bowel movement is there or not. This can help one foster the good habit of having bowel movement at a regular time each day.

3. Be faithful in practising abdominal breathing or massage. This increases secretions and peristalsis in the stomach and intestines and promotes smooth bowel movement.

Treatment:

1. One who finds it difficult to excrete hardened feces may drink a glass (300 to 500 millilitres) of honey water before taking any food each day. This lubricates the intestines and facilitates bowel movement. One may also eat five or six large pitted dates with their peel, raw or steamed.

2. Select one of such herbal preparations as *Ma Zi Ren Wan* (hemp seed pill) or *Wu Ren Wan* (five-kernel pill), both containing oily kernels that facilitate bowel movement. One who does not have strength enough to excrete feces may take *Bu Zhong Yi Qi Wan* (pill for invigorating the spleen and stomach) and *Ren Shen Jian Pi Wan* (ginseng spleen-strengthening pill).

3. Eat bananas frequently. This facilitates bowel

movement, lowers blood pressure and is effective for aged hypertensives with habitual constipation.

4. Bring 30 g of honey with water to a boil and mix an egg into it, beating constantly. Then add sesame oil. Eat a bowl of this every morning.

Obesity

A fat person, in general, is one whose weight exceeds the standard at least by 20 percent, but if the excess is below 30 percent, this is still not considered obese. Only when the excess is above standard by 35 to 40 percent does it make one susceptible to coronary heart disease, diabetes and hypertension. Some people grow fat because of internal secretion disorder or other illnesses. The majority of fat people have simply to blame themselves for overeating.

Prevention:

1. Eat less sugar and animal fat and do more exercises to consume excessive nutriment in the body, preventing it from being transformed into fat.

2. Some become fat hereditarily. Therefore one should take preventive measures as early as possible, and especially in childhood and before climacteric.

Treatment: It is most important to eat less and do more physical exercises. Besides, one may take food therapy or medicine.

1. Boil porridge with fresh or dried lotus leaf. Eat the porridge for ten days. One can lose five kilograms and lower his blood fat.

2. Drink Chinese fat-reducing teas.

Diabetes

Diabetes is a common disease of the middle-aged and elderly. After the age of 40, its incidence rises about 10 percent for every 10 years of age. Typical diabetics are characterized by excessive hunger, thirst and urination, but these symptoms may not be apparent in elderly patients.

Prevention:

1. Eat less sweet food; eat plenty of onions, garlic and hawthorn. This will lower blood fat and sugar and prevent both coronary heart disease and diabetes.

2. Do body-building exercises to avoid becoming fat.

3. When one contracts diabetes, prompt treatment is important to prevent its development.

Treatment: Insulin is often used, but it has severe side effects. Besides, diabetes in the elderly can generally be cured without insulin, by dieting, practising body-building exercises and taking herbal medicines.

1. One should eat plenty of green-leaf vegetables and eat less rice and wheat flour, which contain large amounts of sugar. Abstain from sweets, eat little fat, but eat plenty of vitamins and protein.

2. Take a walk for an hour every morning.

3. Take ginseng alone or boil six g of ginseng and 15 g of Chinese wolfberry into a solution. One dose every day has a remarkable curative effect.

4. Simmer 50 g of the root bark of Chinese wolfberry with one litre of water on low heat to a decoction of 500 millilitres, divided into three doses each day. Meanwhile, take intravenous injection of 100 mg of vitamin C and muscular injection of 100 mg of vitamin B, twice each day. All these should be taken for one full week.

5. There are several food therapies.

Grind 60 g each of black fungus and hyacinth bean into fine powder. Dissolve nine g of the powder in boiling water and drink the solution two or three times a day.

Bring a pig pancreas, three eggs and 60 g of spinach. Slice the pancreas and boil until well-done, beat eggs into it and add fresh spinach. Bring the mixture to a boil and eat the soup with its contents, once each day for ten days.

Eat the tender leaves of cactus as a vegetable, or scrape the thorny skin from the tender leaves, boil and cut them into threds, mixing them with vegetable oil and adding cowpeas and chilli. Sandwich them into thin maize pancakes and take this as a daily meal. This has good effect on lowering blood sugar.

Wash raw Chinese yams and steam in a closed steamer. Separately, boil 30 g each of Chinese wolfberry and the root of Mongolian snakegourd into a soup. Drink the soup while eating 120 g of the cooked Chinese yams. Do this twice each day for a month.

Hypertrophy of Prostate

Hypertrophy of prostate afflicts seven out of ten men between 60 and 70. The prostate gland is an accessory sexual gland through which the urethra also passes. It is located at the outlet of the bladder, and a slight enlargement puts pressure on the bladder, resulting in frequent, dribbling urination, especially at night. If the prostate gland enlarges further, pressure on the urethra restricts urination, resulting in acute retention of urine. The urethra may even be completely blocked so no urine can pass.

Symptoms of hypertrophy will be aggravated by fatigue, alcohol, sexual performance and the common cold.

Prevention:

1. After the age of 40, men should regularly practise propping-scrotum exercises to prevent enlarged pros-

tate.

2. Strike a proper balance between work and rest. Be especially temperate in sexual activity.

3. When symptoms of impotence and nocturnal emission occur along with male sexual decline, prompt treatment is needed to prevent enlarged prostate.

Treatment: One may take medicine in the early stage of the disease. Otherwise he should consider surgery.

1. The disease can be treated with "716 tablets," made with medicinal herbs in Lanzhou.

2. Eat 30 g of well-chewed pumpkin seeds every day. This can both treat enlarged prostate and improve sexual function.

3. Wild chrysanthemum suppository (suppository for anus) is effective on both chronic prostatitis and enlarged prostate.

4. Take food therapy. "Shrimp, sea horse and young chicken" and "double-whip male invigorating soup" can serve as auxiliary treatment. One may also eat frequently fresh shrimps stir-fried with Chinese chives. This treats enlarged prostate and sexual decline.

Sexual Decline

Sexual decline, according to Chinese medical theory, includes male impotence, premature ejaculation and female impotence. Generally speaking, when men exceed the age of 55 to 60, their sexual function gradually declines due to the atrophy and degeneration of their testicles, gradually reducing the secretion of testosterone. Nevertheless, some men in their 80s are still capable of sexual activity. When women reach an age between 45 and 50, their ovaries and reproductive organs begin to atrophy, menstruation gradually becomes irregular and sexual desire gradually declines. In general, women over 60 have no sexual desire.

It is known that reduction in the secretions of sexual glands parallels the aging process. Experiments show that removing testicles results in premature senility in animals. Therefore, delaying decline in sexual organs and sexual function can prolong life.

Prevention: Sexual decline often results from one's unfavourable psychological state and the deterioration of one's general physical conditions.

1. Premature sexual decline is mostly related to over-indulgence in sexual desires in youth and at the prime of life. Consequently, one should be temperate in sexual behaviour at early ages. This is an important preventative of senile sexual decline and also a good way to prevent premature aging.

2. Practise propping-scrotum exercises and other methods of *qigong*.

3. Cultivate diversified interests in music, chess, calligraphy and painting to maintain a lively mental state.

Treatment:

1. Men who suffer from sexual decline can take one of the following medicines: *Qing Chun Bao* (youth treasure), *Hui Chun Bao* (rejuvenating treasure), *Nan Bao* (male treasure), *Zhi Bao San Bian Wan* (triple-whip pill), or Chinese life-preserving wine.

2. Women who suffer from sexual decline can take placenta powder and pills containing wolfberry, chrysanthemum, and glutinous rehmannia.

3. Patients of male sexual decline can take food therapy such as double-whip male-invigorating soup; shrimp, sea horse and young chicken; Chinese wolfberry porridge; knotweed porridge; or caterpillar fungus and sparrow meat prepared thus: First, remove the

feathers and internal organs of five sparrows, wash clean and cut into pieces. Put them in an earthen pot, add water, 10 g of caterpillar fungus and three g of ginger. Stew for two to three hours until the sparrow meat is very well-done.

Climacteric Syndrome

The climacteric syndrome is caused by the degeneration of ovaries in women and of testicles in men. Symptoms are not conspicuous for most men, though some become ill-tempered, impatient, irritable, reticent, unsociable, eccentric or subject to rapid mood changes. General symptons include irritability, insomnia, fatigue, dizziness, headache, memory decline, fluctuations in blood pressure and sexual decline.

Women usually have more apparent symptoms connected with menstruation disorder. They may have a spell of sudden hot flashes and sweating of the face and head, probably followed by irritability, dizziness, palpitation and chills. Such symptoms may recur up to several times each day.

Prevention: Generally speaking, symptoms can be alleviated for women and entirely prevented for men.

1. Most .methods of preventing sexual decline can serve to alleviate climacteric syndrome. Practising *qigong* can maintain the balance of internal secretion.

2. Be forthright, optimistic and broad-minded.

3. Avoid growing fat.

Treatment: Generally, this does not require any treatment because it is a normal physiological process. If the symptoms are too prominent, one can take medicines that treat sexual decline. Women with the menopause syndrome may be helped by the following food therapy. Boil 6 g of liquorice root, 30 g of large dates and 50 g of wheat with water into thick broth and remove the dregs. Take the broth once every morning and evening for a full week.

Senile Dementia

Senile dementia is caused by diffused atrophy of the cerebra in elderly people. Its most prominent symptom is severe memory decline. The patient begins to forget recent events and may proceed, by and by, to the point of forgetting family members, personal experiences and even his own name. When going out, he cannot find the way back home. He becomes unsociable and eccentric, selfish, stubborn, irritable and quarrelsome. In the later stage he gets dull and slow-witted, apathetic and deject-ed, fails to enunciate clearly and garbles speech. Finally, he falls into exhaustion, becomes bed-ridden and can-not attend to himself in daily life.

Prevention: It is of primary importance to use one's brain a great deal.

1. Do not idle away time after retirement. One should continue to study, to use his brain for mental cultivation. This prevents the atrophy of the cerebra.

2. Do not sit alone at home. One should often invite old friends to chat, play chess, and compose or recite poems. Always stay cheerful and open-hearted.

3. Take herbal medicines to nourish the kidneys and the brain. One may eat three to five raw walnuts, walnut porridge or knotweed porridge every morning and evening.

Treatment:

1. It is best for the elderly to live with their children and grandchildren to enjoy family harmony and happi-ness.

2. Take carp head steamed with tubers of elevated

gastrodia, and walnut or sesame porridge frequently.

Senile Lumbago and Leg Pain

Senile lumbago and leg ache are common in the aged. When standing, sitting and walking, one's lumbar vertebrae bear great pressure. With the advance of age, degeneration occurs in the intervertebral discs between the lumbar vertebrae, especially the disc between the fourth and fifth lumbar vertebrae. This involves osteo-hyperplasia of the vertebrae and the growth of spurs on their edges; both stimulate or press against adjoining nerves and cause chronic lumbago and leg ache.

Osteoporosis may also cause chronic lumbago and leg ache. When it grows severe, spinal compression fracture may occur, suddenly aggravating lumbago and making the patient unable to straighten the lower back.

Prevention:

1. Do not sit, stand or walk for long periods of time. Practise *taijiquan* and massage to limber up the lower back.

2. Elderly people with general weaknesses may take herbal medicines to nourish the kidneys and strengthen the waist. One may choose tablets for strengthening the kidneys produced by Shanghai No. 3 Herbal Medicine Factory and tiger-bone wine produced by Guiyang Herbal Medicine Factory.

Treatment: Choose from the following methods if the symptoms are not severe. Otherwise the patient should go to hospital.

1. Hot compress on the afflicted location to alleviate pain. Musk-and-tiger-bone paster or dog-skin plaster can also be applied.

2. Take over a long period osteohyperplasia tablets made by Jilin Herbal Medicine Factory, lumbago tablets

made by Hangzhou Huqingyutang Pharmaceutical Factory and spur pills made by Shanxi Provincial Research Institute of Traditional Chinese Medicine and Pharmacology.

3. Apply herbal pad to the waist. Grind 15 g each of radix aconiti, radix aconiti Kusnezoffii and herba asari; 12 g each of cassia twig and cinnamon; 10 g of clove; 30 g each of rhizoma sparganii, rhizoma zedoariae and the rhizome of nutgrass flatsedge and 5 g of borneol together into fine powder to make a small herbal pad, two to three centimetres thick, 25 centimetres long and 20 centimetres wide. Place tightly against the waist when lying down or fasten around the waist at other times. This can warm up the channels, promote blood circulation and ease pain.

Cervical Vertebra Disease

It is frequent and recurring among the elderly. With advancing age, the lower section of one's cervical vertebrae is liable to degenerate. Osteohyperplasia presses against the root of spinal nerves and causes pain in the neck, back and arms. Sometimes the pain radiates along the upper limbs to the fingers, which become numb or feel like electrified. The pain increases when the head turns to a certain position and eases when the head returns to the front. Sometimes the neck becomes stiff as if cramped during sleep. If there is a large spur behind the vertebrae, it may press against the spinal cord, numbing the hands and causing clumsy, unsteady steps. Sometimes a spur grows on the side of the cervical vertebrae and presses against the vertebral artery that supplies blood to the brain, so that when one's head turns, symptoms of insuficent blood supply will appear such as dizziness, headache and affected vision.

Prevention: Avoid working at the desk or lifting the head to watch television or films over a long period. One should limber up the neck at one hour intervals so neck muscles and ligaments are flexed and rested. The pillow should be neither too high nor too low; a thickness of 10 centimetres is recommended.

Treatment:

1. Massage the cervical vertebrae to alleviate pain.

2. Take herbal preparations to promote blood circulation and limber up the tendons and joints. One may choose from *Gu Zhi Zeng Sheng Pian* (osteohyperplasia tablets), *Tian Ma Wan* (elevated gastrodia pills) or *Yu Feng Ning Xin Pian* (mind-calming tablets with radix puerariae as the main ingredient).

3. Herbal pillow therapy. Grind 200 g of rhizoma ligustici and 150 g of rhizoma seu radix notopterygii into powder and stuff into a pillowcase of cotton cloth or silk for use as a pillow to ease pain and promote blood circulation.

Senile Deafness

Generally, one's hearing begins to decline between age 40 and 50, and some finally become totally deaf. However, there are centenarians who retain normal hearing all their lives.

Senile deafness is often accompanied by tinnitus. Senility brings physiological degenerative changes to the ears. The patient feels as if there were cicada chirping in his ears. Noise, smoking, alcohol or cardiovascular diseases can accelerate the development of deafness and tinnitus.

Prevention: It is absolutely necessary to take preventative cautions, for treatment of the disease is fairly difficult.

1. Maintain a quiet environment and avoid the stimulus of noise over a long period.

2. Abstain from smoking and excessive alcohol, for nicotine and alcohol can damage hearing nerves.

3. Take precautions against using streptomycin and kanamycin, both of which damage hearing nerves.

4. Massage the ears to improve blood supply there.

Treatment: This does not rely mainly on medicines. But one may take herbal preparations for nourishing the kidneys.

Senile Cataract

Senile cataract is the main disease that causes blindness in the elderly. It occurs when albumin in the lens becomes denatured. In the early stage vision blurs, with dot or cloud-like opacities and illusory or double vision, such as seeing two moons. When cataract develops fully, total blindness occurs.

Prevention: Once cataracts occur they cannot be cured, so it is of primary importance to prevent their appearances.

1. Massage the eyes frequently. Do not watch television over a long time period by looking directly at the screen.

2. Cataracts may be a complication of diabetes, which therefore must be treated without delay.

Treatment: Medicines may help in the incipient stage, but the patient must resort to surgery in late stages.

1. As cataracts begin, one may apply *Jing Ming* (eyebrightening) eyedrops, *Li Ming* (vision-benefitting) eyedrops and vitamin B2 eyedrops, four times each day. One may also take vitamins B1, B2 and C orally, or *Shi Hu Ye Guang Wan* (pills containing the stem of noble dendrobium) and *Ming Mu Di Huang Wan* (glutinous

rehmannia pills).

2. If the cataracts have matured, the patient can take surgery of traditional methods at any traditional Chinese medicine hospitals in China.

Cancer

After the age of 40 the human immunity system gradually declines, with increasing possibility of the occurrence of cancer. Therefore, the likelihood of cancer rises after one passes the age of 40, and it accelerates as one enters old age. Many tissues and organs of the human body are vulnerable to the disease, so cancer has many varieties.

Prevention: It is still difficult today to treat cancer in its late stages, so stress should be put on prevention. It has been discovered that many varieties of cancer are closely related to chronic inflammations, virus infections, and mechanical, chemical or radioactive stimuli over a long period. Besides, cancer can also find its way in by the mouth.

1. Be forthright and cheerful and avoid fatigue.

2. Remove strange, black moles.

3. Prevent and treat without delay hepatitis, especially type B hepatitis.

4. Remove hysteromyoma and treat cervical erosion without delay.

5. Prevent and treat stomach ulcers, atrophic gastritis, and constipation.

6. Abstain from smoking and be moderate with alcohol.

7. Diversify diet and do not be too particular about food. Eat less salt, for salty food can lead to esophagal cancer.

8. Do not eat food that is scorched or mouldy.

Mouldy food contains aflatoxin, a highly carcinogenic substance. Avoid smoked or preserved food. Do not eat food that is too hot, hard or peppery to prevent inflammation of the esophagus and stomach.

9. Do not expose oneself to scorching sunlight or radioactive substance.

10. Avoid inhaling strange gases, especially wastes from factories which are highly carcinogenic.

11. Those with low immunity may take medicinal herbs such as Chinese wolfberry, glossy ganoderma (*Ganoderma lucidum*), membraneous milkvetch, ginseng and mushroom.

Treatment: No specific medicine is available, but food therapy may prevent cancer and have some relieving effect.

1. Mushroom improves the immunity function of the human body against cancer.

2. Animal liver contains cancer-inhibiting substances such as vitamin A, zinc and selenium.

3. Eating food rich in vitamin A such as tomato, carrot and edible sea weeds can help prevent lung, liver and colon cancers.

4. Cucumber contains cucurbitacin C, which can inhibit cancer as well as prevent sugar from transforming into fat in the human body.

5. Turnip contains enzymes that forestall the cancer-inducing effect of amine nitrite. Lignin in turnips can improve the vitality of giant phagocites, enabling them to absorb cancerous cells.

6. Eat garlic, bean sprouts, lettuce, cabbage, pumpkin and peas.

7. Drink cow's and goat's milk. Eat sword bean, goose blood and tremella. Eat food rich in protein such as soy

beans, fish and lean meat.

8. Royal jelly strengthens the immunity function of human body.

9. All varieties of tea are effective in cancer prevention, especially Wulong tea.

10. Take food therapy. Eat eight-treasure chicken soup and multi-herb nourishing soup to improve immunity function. Eat duck steamed with Chinese caterpillar fungus to treat lung cancer and lean meat stewed with sealwort to treat gastric cancer.

Traditional Chinese Therapeutic Exercises and Techniques

Atlas of Therapeutic Motion for Treatment and Health
—A Guide to Traditional Chinese Massage and Exercise Therapy

Traditional Chinese Therapeutic Exercises
Standing Pole

Chinese Single Broadsword
A Primer of Basic Skills and Performance Routines for Practitioners

14-Series Sinew-Transforming Exercises

Infantile *Tuina* Therapy

Eating Your Way to Health
Dietotherapy in Traditional Chinese Medicine

Keep Fit the Chinese Way

Meridian Qigong

Taiji Qigong
Twenty-eight Steps

The Mystery of Longevity

图书在版编目(CIP)数据

长寿之谜:英文/刘正才编著
—北京:外文出版社,1990 (1996 重印)
ISBN 7 – 119 – 01251 – 7

Ⅰ.长… Ⅱ.刘… Ⅲ.长寿 – 保健 – 方法 – 英文 Ⅳ.R161.7

中国版本图书馆 CIP 数据核字 (96) 第 14662 号

责任编辑 蔡希芹 周奎杰
封面设计 蔡 荣

长寿之谜

刘正才 著

＊

©外文出版社
外文出版社出版
(中国北京百万庄大街 24 号)
邮政编码 100037
北京外文印刷厂印刷
中国国际图书贸易总公司发行
(中国北京车公庄西路 35 号)
北京邮政信箱第 399 号 邮政编码 100044
1990 年(34 开)第 1 版
1996 年第 1 版第 3 次印刷
(英)
ISBN 7 – 119 – 01251 – 7 /R·49(外)
01350
14 – E – 2421P